Freeing Yourself from Emotional DependencyA Journey of Awareness, Autonomy, and Love

Introduction

- Introduction to the concept of emotional dependency.
- Why it is important to talk about emotional dependency today.
- The objectives of the book: awareness, understanding, and personal growth.
- A brief overview of the topics that will be covered in the various chapters.
- An invitation to the reader to reflect on themselves and their relationship experiences.

Part 1: Understanding Emotional Dependency

Chapter 1: What is Emotional Dependency?

- The psychological definition of emotional dependency.
- The difference between healthy love and emotional dependency.
- The confusion between romantic love and the obsessive need to be loved.
- The history of the concept of emotional dependency in modern psychology.

Chapter 2: The Causes of Emotional Dependency

- Psychological factors: low self-esteem, fear of abandonment.
- Cultural and social factors: models of love in media and families.
- The influence of childhood: relationships with parents and attachment figures.
- Emotional wounds: trauma and lack of affection.

Chapter 3: The Dynamics of Dependency in Relationships

- The main characteristics of an emotionally dependent relationship.
- The roles of victim and perpetrator in toxic relationships.
- Cycles of dependency: attraction, idealization, disillusionment, and dependency.
- Codependency: when both partners are emotionally dependent.

- The role of gratitude and forgiveness towards oneself.

Chapter 14: Relationships and Healthy Love

- How to recognize a healthy and fulfilling relationship.
- Differences between romantic love and dependent love.
- Mature relationships: individual and couple growth.
- Learning to live love in a free and authentic way.

Chapter 15: The Future of Your Emotional Life

- How to maintain emotional balance over time.
- Continuing the path of personal growth: life as a constant evolution.
- The freedom to love without being dependent.
- The importance of staying aware and vigilant about your emotions.

Introduction to the Concept of Emotional Dependency

Imagine a river flowing peacefully, nourishing everything it encounters along its path: trees, flowers, animals. However, this river has a source that continually feeds it, a secret and hidden place from which its crystal-clear waters spring. If that source were to dry up, the river would begin to dry up as well, eventually becoming an arid bed, incapable of giving life. Emotional dependency is something similar. It is like a river that does not have its own autonomous source but continually feeds off an external source, seeking in the other what it should find within itself. It is the urgent need to feel complete, loved, and valued, which ties us in an almost visceral way to another person, making us believe that without them, we are destined for emptiness and meaninglessness.

Emotional dependency is a state of the soul that many confuse with love, a feeling disguised as a bond but, in reality, hides an invisible chain. It is that pervasive feeling that drives us to place the other at the center of our emotional world, to sacrifice our needs and desires out of fear of being abandoned. Our identity dissolves, merging with that of the partner, in a dance where fear and desire alternate, and control and submission become the main steps.

This concept, although so common and widespread, is difficult to recognize within a relationship. Emotional dependency hides behind seemingly normal gestures and feelings that are sometimes exalted by culture, such as jealousy or exclusivity. It feeds on unrealistic expectations, idealizations, and the belief that love must necessarily be painful or sacrificial. The image of romantic love that is often presented to us is filled with lovers willing to do anything to stay together, even at the cost of losing themselves. But in this scenario, love turns into need, into obsession. And it is here that emotional dependency sneaks in.

Those who are victims of it are not aware, at least initially, of how much this dynamic consumes them from within. They live in the belief that their worth depends on the gaze of the other, that without that person, happiness could not exist. Every small inattention, every sign of distance is experienced as a threat, a confirmation of a looming danger: loneliness. It is an ancestral fear, that of abandonment, rooted in experiences often forgotten or never processed, but it manifests forcefully in adult relationships. Thus, one enters a cycle of anxious attachment, where the dependent person becomes incapable of finding peace or serenity without the constant reassurance of the other.

But emotional dependency is not limited to a relationship between two people. It becomes a lens through which the world is viewed, influencing every relationship and self-perception. The emotionally dependent person may live an apparently normal life, but inside they feel perpetually empty, as if a fundamental piece for their happiness is missing. And so begins the desperate search for who or what can fill that void. Often, this search leads to nothing stable or lasting. Paradoxically, the more one tries to fill their need through the other, the more the sense of inadequacy deepens.

What makes emotional dependency so complex is its link with the concept of love. So, how can we distinguish it from true love? How can we recognize when a relationship is nurturing and reciprocal, rather than unbalanced and stifling? Healthy love is based on freedom, respect, and autonomy. It is a natural flow of emotions and exchanges, in which both parties grow and enrich themselves without losing their identity. Emotional dependency, on the other hand, blocks this flow. It focuses on possession, control, and the anxiety of losing the other, fueling dynamics of power and submission.

In this introduction, we begin a journey of discovery towards greater awareness. We will analyze where this form of dependency originates, what its psychological roots are, and what strategies we can adopt to break the cycle of dependency. Because, although today it may seem impossible to live without that bond, the reality is that true freedom and true love are born from an inner balance, from a source that springs within us and not from outside. This book is intended to be a guide for those who want to rediscover themselves, for those tired of living relationships based on fear and lack, and who want to learn how to build authentic relationships, based on mutual love and autonomy.

Whether you are already aware of your emotional dependency or are just discovering it now, the path to emotional freedom is possible. And the first step is right here, in understanding this concept that is as complex as it is necessary to explore.

Why It Is Important to Talk About Emotional Dependency Today We live in an age where connection seems to be at our fingertips. Social media, instant messaging, and video calls give us the illusion of always being close, always in touch with the world and others. Yet, never before has humanity had to deal with such deep loneliness, hidden behind the glowing screen of our smartphone, concealed behind the perfect smiles we post on Instagram. In this digital reality, paradoxically, emotional dependency finds fertile ground to take root and thrive, as love and attention have become commodities, measured in "likes" and virtual red hearts. Talking about emotional dependency today is not only a psychological urgency but a social and cultural necessity.

Contemporary society has built a myth around love, an unattainable ideal of emotional perfection that pushes us to seek in the other not only love but also our identity and worth. We are taught that being alone is synonymous with failure, that romantic love is the pinnacle of happiness, and that without a partner, we are incomplete. This message surrounds us everywhere: in films, songs, advertisements, and popular stories. Emotional dependency feeds on this culture that exalts love as the solution to all problems, portraying life without an "other" as meaningless. But what is not said is that love, when it becomes an obsessive need, turns into a shadow that suffocates the individual.

Talking about emotional dependency today is necessary because more and more people, unknowingly, live in toxic and stifling relationships, convinced that this is normal, that love must be suffering, sacrifice, or that jealousy and possession are tangible proofs of the feeling. Often, we settle for relationships that drain our souls for fear of loneliness, accepting devastating emotional compromises just to avoid being alone with ourselves. The subtle message that has insinuated itself into collective culture is that loneliness is an enemy to be fought, a shame to be hidden, and this fuels unbalanced emotional dynamics, where we lose touch with our deep inner self.

Today, more than ever, talking about emotional dependency is essential to break these invisible chains that imprison thousands of people. In a context where self-esteem is fragile, often measured based on external standards, and where human relationships have become superficial, the importance of healthy and autonomous love is crucial. Emotional dependency makes us believe that the other is the key to our happiness, but this belief hides a trap: the conviction that we are not enough on our own, that we are worthless without the gaze of the other to legitimize our existence.

Today, mental health and inner well-being are increasingly discussed, yet emotional dependency remains an underrated, if not ignored, issue. And yet, it represents a deep emotional wound that affects people of all ages, genders, and cultural backgrounds. In a world where everything seems accelerated, even relationships have become "disposable," and yet emotional dependency often prolongs relationships that are already over, keeping people chained to situations that drain their energy, preventing them from evolving. Addressing this issue means offering people the opportunity to understand that true love, above all, must be born within themselves, from self-understanding and the acceptance of their uniqueness.

It is not just an individual issue. Talking about emotional dependency today also has collective value, as the dynamics of power and submission that arise in toxic relationships also impact broader social structures. Emotional dependency often fuels forms of control and manipulation, which can lead to emotional or physical abuse. In a society that promotes individual empowerment, recognizing emotional dependency is an essential step in giving people back their strength, teaching them that true power does not lie in controlling the other but in the ability to love in a free and reciprocal way.

Today, many people live behind a mask, showing the world a façade of confidence, but inside they harbor a sense of dissatisfaction and emptiness. This emptiness is often filled with relationships that offer temporary fulfillment but do not lead to personal growth. Talking about emotional dependency means addressing the issue of inner emptiness and the need for self-completion. It means recognizing that happiness cannot be given by someone else but must be built with patience and dedication within oneself. Only once we have found our own completeness can we enter into healthy relationships, where the other is not a reflection of our worth but a companion with whom to share a journey of mutual growth.

In a rapidly changing world, where uncertainties and fears are the order of the day, talking about emotional dependency is an act of courage. It is an invitation to rediscover the value of individuality and to learn to be happy even alone, without having to depend emotionally on another. Because true love, the kind that frees and elevates us, can only exist when we are free to be ourselves, without chains, without fears.

Today, more than ever, we need to remember that the true relationship begins with the one we build with ourselves. Talking about emotional dependency means shining a light on the shadowy areas of our hearts and inviting each of us to rediscover the beauty of a love that is not a need, but a choice. A conscious and free choice.

The Objectives of the Book: Awareness, Understanding, and Personal Growth This book was written with a specific purpose: to be a guiding light for those immersed in the darkness of emotional dependency, leading them toward new awareness, deep and authentic understanding, and ultimately, a journey of personal growth that not only frees them from the invisible chains of dependency but also leads to a more authentic and free form of love. Every word, every chapter, has been designed as an invitation to reflect, to delve into the depths of the soul, and to emerge with new inner strength.

Awareness: The First Step Toward Freedom Awareness is the starting point, the awakening. It is like the first ray of sunlight filtering through a forgotten open window, illuminating corners of ourselves that had remained in the shadows until that moment. We often live our relationships on autopilot, conditioned by models we have internalized without realizing it, driven by needs we cannot name. We are so consumed by the urgency to be loved that we never stop to ask why, to explore what lies behind that insatiable thirst for love that consumes us.

This book aims to help the reader do just that: stop and look inside. Awareness is a revolutionary act; it is the ability to observe one's thoughts, emotions, and behaviors without judgment, but with profound honesty. For those suffering from emotional dependency, this step is crucial because it is easy to get lost in the maze of one's emotions without having a map showing the way out. Being aware of one's emotional dependency means recognizing the mechanisms that drive us to constantly seek validation and reassurance from others; it means observing the dynamics of control and submission that often manifest in our relationships.

Awareness, however, is not just observation. It is also the courage to accept what we discover. It is not easy to admit that we emotionally depend on someone else or that we have built our self-esteem on the fragile ground of others' approval. But only through this acceptance, only through this awareness, can a process of transformation begin. The book will guide the reader on this inner journey, providing tools and reflections to explore the roots of their dependency and awaken a new vision of themselves and their relationships.

Understanding: A Journey Into the Depths of the Soul If awareness is the awakening, understanding is the journey that follows. It is a deeper process that requires time and patience. Understanding means uncovering the hidden causes behind our behaviors and desires. Emotional dependency, after all, does not arise out of nowhere. It is the result of a complex web of past experiences, unhealed wounds, and unmet needs. Often, the roots of this dependency lie in childhood, in relationships with attachment figures who failed to provide us with security, unconditional love, or emotional presence. Other times, emotional dependency is the product of trauma or a history of abandonment that has deeply shaped our view of love and relationships.

The book aims to lead the reader through a path of inner exploration, helping them understand not only the causes of their dependency but also the dynamics it generates. Understanding also means becoming aware that emotional dependency is not a life sentence but a learned behavior that can be unlearned. It is like looking at one's heart through a magnifying glass, discovering all the nuances and details that had previously remained hidden.

Therefore, understanding is also about self-empathy. It is the moment when we stop judging ourselves for our weaknesses and start seeing our story with new eyes, full of compassion and respect. Understanding one's dependency means recognizing it for what it is: perhaps a clumsy attempt to protect oneself from the pain of loneliness, from the feeling of inadequacy. But it also means learning to recognize that there is another way to live and love, a healthier and more fulfilling way.

Personal Growth: The Awakening of Authentic Love The third and final goal of this book is perhaps the most ambitious, but also the most rewarding: personal growth. Talking about emotional dependency does not just mean understanding the problem, but most importantly, embarking on a path of transformation, an evolution toward a more authentic and free form of love. Personal growth, in this context, is a process of reclaiming oneself, rediscovering one's identity and inner strength. It is learning to live relationships not as a refuge from loneliness, but as an encounter between two complete, autonomous individuals, capable of loving each other without losing themselves.

Growth means learning to set healthy boundaries, to say "no" when necessary, to recognize one's needs and meet them without relying solely on the other. It means accepting that happiness is not something that comes from outside, but something that is built within, day by day, through small acts of self-care and love. Personal growth is not a linear path: it consists of steps forward and backward, of discoveries and moments of difficulty. But it is also a journey that leads to greater emotional freedom, to more balanced and satisfying relationships.

The book will provide practical tools for this journey of growth: reflection exercises, mindfulness techniques, suggestions for improving self-esteem, and strategies for building healthier relationships. The goal is to help the reader develop a new vision of love, no longer based on dependency, but on sharing and reciprocity. Growth also means learning to accept imperfection, in oneself and in others, without trying to change or control those around us. It means understanding that true love is not possession but freedom, that it is not fueled by need but by conscious choice.

Conclusion: A Journey of Rebirth Awareness, understanding, and personal growth are the three pillars on which this book is based. They are the goals the reader can pursue through its pages, not as distant and unattainable destinations, but as milestones on a path of rebirth. The journey from emotional dependency to authentic love is an inner journey, full of reflections and discoveries, challenges, and triumphs. But it is also a necessary journey because only by freeing ourselves from the chains of dependency can we truly experience the joy of loving and being loved in a healthy and fulfilling way.

This book is an invitation to look inside with honesty and compassion, to recognize one's wounds, and to work on healing them. It is a guide for those who want not only to understand themselves but also to transform their lives and relationships, bringing greater authenticity and freedom to their way of loving. And, above all, it is a message of hope: emotional dependency can be overcome, and beyond its shadows lies a love that is not tied to fear but to true freedom.

A Brief Overview of the Topics Covered in the Various Chapters The journey we are about to embark on through these pages is a deep dive into the labyrinths of the mind and heart, an exploration that will touch the most intimate strings of the human being. This book, like a discreet but present companion on the road, will accompany the reader on the arduous path that leads from emotional dependency to emotional freedom. Through the various chapters, we will address the themes that will help us understand the roots of this form of dependency, its manifestations, and, most importantly, the ways to overcome it and reach a more balanced, authentic, and autonomous emotional dimension.

Part I: Understanding Emotional Dependency The first step on this journey will be to understand what emotional dependency really is. In the initial chapters, we will approach the topic from a psychological perspective, clearly distinguishing healthy love from love distorted by the need for possession and control. We will understand how emotional dependency arises from complex dynamics rooted in the past, often in childhood, when our capacity to love and be loved is shaped by our first significant relationships.

We will explore the deep causes of emotional dependency, shedding light on the soul's wounds that push us to seek in the other what is missing inside. We will analyze how the fear of abandonment, low self-esteem, and emotional emptiness become fertile ground for developing a distorted emotional relationship, where the need for affirmation and reassurance replaces genuine love. This will allow us to illuminate the hidden mechanisms that fuel dependency, giving us a clearer and more conscious vision of our inner world.

Part II: Recognizing Dependency in Relationships After exploring the causes and dynamics of emotional dependency, we will focus on a practical analysis of the signs that may indicate a dysfunctional relationship. We will learn to recognize the warning signs: that constant sense of anxiety that grips us when the partner is away for even a short time, the compulsive need to control and know where they are, the constant sacrifice of our happiness for the other, and that oppressive feeling of being incomplete without them. Recognizing these signs is the first step toward liberation, as it allows us to clearly identify what is keeping us trapped in the cage of dependency.

In the following chapters, we will examine the different forms of emotional dependency that can manifest in romantic relationships, but also in family and professional settings. We will see how emotional dependency can take on various shades, from anxious attachment in a romantic relationship to emotional submission in a parental relationship, to the codependency that often develops between people bound by strong emotional ties but unable to establish healthy boundaries.

Part III: The Psychological Roots of Dependency Digging even deeper, we will explore the psychological roots of emotional dependency, focusing on two key aspects: attachment style and self-esteem. Through the lens of attachment theory, we will discover how our early relationships with caregivers influence our way of relating as adults. Insecure attachment styles, such as anxious or avoidant attachment, can predispose us to develop emotional dependency in adulthood, creating a constant fear of being abandoned or, conversely, the tendency to avoid intimacy for fear of rejection.

Self-esteem plays a crucial role in this pattern. We will delve into how a negative perception of oneself can drive us to seek validation from others. We will examine the link between low self-esteem and emotional dependency and reflect on how strengthening one's self-esteem can be an essential step in breaking the cycle of dependency. Finally, we will understand how the fear of loneliness fuels the obsessive need to have someone by our side, making it difficult, if not impossible, to find fulfillment in our own company.

Part IV: The Path to Freedom Once we understand the nature of emotional dependency and recognize its signs, we will turn to the heart of our journey: the healing process. In the chapters dedicated to this topic, we will address the challenges of leaving a toxic or codependent relationship. We will analyze the fears that hold us back, the emptiness we fear, and learn practical strategies to strengthen our emotional autonomy.

The path to freedom is not easy, but it is profoundly liberating. We will discover how to establish healthy emotional boundaries, how to build a support network to help us through the most challenging moments, and how to use practices like mindfulness to ground ourselves in the present, learning to recognize and manage our emotions without being overwhelmed by them. Through practical examples, therapeutic techniques, and self-assessment tools, we will be guided toward a new awareness and the construction of a stronger and more independent emotional identity.

Part V: Loving Autonomously and Consciously Finally, in the concluding chapters of the book, we will explore what it means to love in a healthy and autonomous way. We will discover that true love is not a cage but a bridge between two people who choose to walk together while remaining complete individuals. We will analyze the characteristics of a balanced relationship based on mutual respect, trust, and open communication. We will see how healthy love does not require destructive sacrifices but is instead a force that enriches both partners, allowing each to grow and realize themselves as individuals.

Loving autonomously also means loving oneself. In the final chapters, we will learn the importance of self-care and self-compassion. We will discover that only when we are capable of loving and accepting ourselves can we truly love the other without dependency or fear. The book will end with an invitation to cultivate authentic love, one that is not fueled by need but by choice, freedom, and mutual respect.

An Invitation to Reflect on Yourself and Your Relationship ExperienceBefore continuing our journey through these pages, I invite you to pause for a moment and turn your gaze inward. Imagine looking at yourself in a mirror, but not just any mirror: a mirror of the soul, capable of reflecting not only your outer image but also the intricate web of your emotions, deepest thoughts, and desires. This mirror is here to show you who you really are, beyond the masks you wear daily, beyond the roles you have grown accustomed to playing in your relationships.

Take a moment and think about the relationships you have experienced or are currently experiencing. Perhaps you have loved intensely, given everything of yourself, and placed your heart in someone else's hands. But have you ever asked yourself what you were truly seeking in that love? Were you looking for a refuge from loneliness? Were you seeking validation to feel worthy, to feel like you mattered? Have you ever felt that, without that person, your world might collapse, as if love were an anchor, an indispensable lifeline to avoid drowning in emptiness?

Reflect for a moment on your relationship experiences. Has there been a time when you felt you were losing yourself for the other person? Have you ever accepted compromises that caused you pain just to maintain the bond? Perhaps you ignored your own needs, dreams, and deepest desires because you feared that if you asked for something for yourself, love would disappear. Or, conversely, you may have tried to control the other, to keep them close to you at all costs, so as not to lose that source of security and affection that seemed to be the only thing giving you value.

This is the moment to reflect on these dynamics. There is no judgment here, only a gentle invitation to explore with honesty. Every relationship offers a lesson, even those that have hurt us or made us feel trapped. But to learn from these experiences, we must look at them with new eyes, in a different light: the light of awareness.

Think about the times when you felt you weren't enough and sought validation from others' gazes. Think about those sleepless nights, spent wondering what more you could have done, what you could have changed to keep the person who was slipping away from you. Or think about that feeling of emptiness you felt when the other was distant, an emptiness that seemed unbearable and that you desperately tried to fill.

It is possible that, in those moments, you were not living love, but emotional dependency. It is a difficult thought to accept, I know. We have been taught to believe that love must be all-consuming, that loving means giving everything, even at the cost of losing oneself. But true love, the kind that frees, does not ask you to lose yourself, does not ask you to sacrifice your happiness or abandon yourself for the other. Authentic love is a dance between two autonomous souls who choose to walk together but without needing to cling to each other out of fear of falling.

So, I invite you to reflect: what kind of love have you experienced so far? What dynamics have repeated themselves in your life? Have you more often felt free or trapped in your relationships? Have you sought the other out of fear of being alone or out of a sincere desire to share your life? And above all, have you ever asked yourself what it truly means to love yourself?

This book will not give you easy answers or immediate solutions. But it will help you ask the right questions. It will accompany you on a journey of discovery, a journey where you will be able to explore the roots of your emotions, your fears, and your hopes. And it will be through this reflection that you will begin to transform the way you live love, letting go of the chains of emotional dependency and opening yourself to a healthier, more balanced, and above all, freer form of relationship.

This reflection is not just about the past or the present, but also the future. Think about the relationships you want to live from now on. Imagine a love that does not suffocate you but allows you to breathe. A love that is not based on the fear of losing but on the joy of sharing. A love where your happiness does not depend on the other but arises from within you, like an inexhaustible source. This is the love you deserve, and this is the love you can aspire to.

The path ahead is not easy. Emotional dependency is a deep dynamic, rooted in life experiences and emotional wounds that we often carry within us without realizing it. But it is possible to heal; it is possible to transform these dynamics, and this book will be a guide, a beacon illuminating the path. It all starts here, with this sincere reflection on who you are, what you desire, and how you want to live your relationships.

Take the time to listen to yourself, to be honest with yourself. And remember, this is not a journey you have to face alone. These pages were written for you, to accompany you step by step, offering you tools for awareness and understanding. But the most important step is the courage to look within and recognize that, whatever your story may be, you deserve a love that never makes you feel less than who you are. A love that is not dependency but a conscious and authentic choice.

Part 1: Understanding Emotional Dependency

Chapter 1

What is Emotional Dependency?

Emotional dependency is like an invisible thread that ties us tightly to another person, but not in that peaceful and reciprocal way that defines healthy love. Instead, it's more like a taut rope that keeps us bound by the fear of being abandoned, driving us to sacrifice our emotional freedom, desires, and sometimes even our dignity, just to avoid the terrifying emptiness we dread. It's the illusion that the other person is the only source of happiness, the only light that guides our path, and without them, we would feel lost, adrift, and worthless.

This form of dependency, unlike authentic love, does not arise from the conscious choice to share one's life with another individual, but from a visceral need, an obsession to be constantly reassured, loved, and accepted. It's as if the emotional dependent's soul were a barren land that, instead of finding nourishment in its own resources, desperately waits for external rain, without which it fears it cannot survive. Emotional dependency feeds on this primordial fear: the fear of loneliness, rejection, of feeling invisible or not enough.

When you are emotionally dependent, the other person becomes the gravitational center of your existence. Your emotions, moods, and daily decisions—all are shaped and conditioned by the partner's mood and actions. Personal happiness no longer depends on internal satisfaction but solely on the other person's approval and presence. If they smile at us, we feel alive; if they ignore us, we feel destroyed. It's like being suspended on a thin wire, at the mercy of every small movement or change from the other person, incapable of maintaining emotional balance independently.

In emotional dependency, love turns into need. You no longer love the other person for who they are, but for how they make you feel. The other becomes a mirror in which you constantly seek validation of your worth. It is a conditional love, where every gesture, every word, every moment together is imbued with an unconscious desire to receive something in return: the assurance of being loved, the certainty of not being left alone. In this way, the relationship stops being a space for growth and becomes an emotional prison.

Emotional dependency comes in many shades. It manifests in different ways depending on the person and the relationship, but some traits are universal. The first is self-sacrifice. The emotionally dependent person tends to place the needs and desires of the other above their own, often to the point of erasing themselves, giving up dreams, ambitions, and even personal values just to avoid losing the relationship. The constant thought is: "If I don't do what the other wants, I'll lose them." This fear drives every decision, leading to a form of emotional submission that gradually erodes one's identity.

Another defining feature of emotional dependency is obsessive jealousy. The person living in this form of dependency feels a constant need to control the other, to know what they are doing, who they are with, and what they are thinking. Every gesture or behavior that suggests even the slightest emotional distance is experienced as an existential threat. Jealousy becomes a defense mechanism against the fear of rejection, but at the same time, it fuels a vicious cycle of insecurity, mistrust, and conflict.

Behind emotional dependency often lies deep insecurity, a rooted belief of not being enough or not deserving love. This insecurity is the seed from which dependency grows, because someone who does not feel complete within themselves will constantly seek to fill that void through another. Their self-esteem becomes inseparably tied to the partner's approval and affection, and without it, they feel lost and worthless.

But how does emotional dependency begin? How can someone come to feel that their happiness depends entirely on someone else? The answer lies in past experiences, in unresolved emotional wounds that often trace back to childhood. Attachment theory, for example, teaches us that the relationships we develop with our parents or caregivers shape how we love and relate as adults. If, as children, we were exposed to unstable relationships, if we experienced abandonment or emotional inconsistency, it's likely that we will develop an insecure attachment style as adults, leading us to constantly seek emotional reassurance to fill unresolved emotional gaps.

In other words, emotional dependency is a response to unmet emotional needs. It is an often unconscious attempt to compensate for an inner void through another. But it is also a path that, unfortunately, leads to suffering, because no one else, no matter how loving and present, can fully fill our gaps. Only we can heal those wounds, only we can learn to be enough for ourselves, to nourish our soul without relying on an external source.

Yet, those who live with emotional dependency often feel trapped in a cycle that seems impossible to break. The more they seek security and stability in the other, the more insecure and unstable they feel, because the source of their happiness lies outside of their control. Every time the other distances themselves, even briefly, that sense of emptiness surges back powerfully, leaving them feeling fragile and powerless.

But there is a way out, a path toward emotional freedom. The first step is awareness: recognizing your emotional dependency, accepting that it exists and that it is a dynamic that is depriving you of the chance to experience authentic love. Only with this awareness can you begin working on yourself, learning to build your self-esteem, recognize your own needs, and find an inner balance that doesn't rely solely on the other person.

Emotional dependency may seem like a prison with no escape, but the truth is that the keys to freedom lie within us. This book aims to offer you one of those keys, a light to illuminate the path toward healthier love, one that thrives on sharing and freedom, not need. Because true love is not dependency, but a meeting between two people who choose to love each other without losing themselves.

Psychological Definition of Emotional Dependency

Emotional dependency is a psychological condition rooted in an individual's emotional and relational sphere. It is a complex dynamic where the need for love, approval, and external validation becomes so pervasive that it erases, or at least compromises, personal autonomy and emotional balance. It manifests as a form of pathological attachment to another person, where affection and love are confused with possession and control, and where one's very existence seems to depend on the other's presence, attention, and reassurance.

Psychologically, emotional dependency can be considered a form of behavioral addiction, in some ways similar to substance addiction. Just as a drug addict cannot live without their daily fix, the emotionally dependent person constantly seeks validation and attention from their partner, without which they feel emotionally distressed. It's not just a simple desire to be loved or appreciated, which is natural and human, but a compulsive and uncontrollable need that dominates the individual's life, preventing them from living peacefully without the other.

From a psychological standpoint, emotional dependency can be described as a state of inner emptiness, a void that the individual tries to fill through their relationship with another. This void often stems from past emotional wounds, unresolved traumas, or unsatisfactory childhood relationships, resulting in an inability to find value, security, and love within oneself. The emotionally dependent person does not perceive themselves as complete but sees the other as their "half," an indispensable part without which they cannot exist in an authentic and fulfilling way. The other becomes the emotional center of their life, the primary, if not exclusive, source of their well-being.

In emotional dependency, the individual unconsciously sacrifices their identity to meet the needs and expectations of the other, hoping this will guarantee them love and emotional stability. Their self-esteem is so tied to the relationship that any sign of distance, real or perceived, is experienced as an existential threat. In this sense, emotional dependency is characterized by anxious attachment: the emotionally dependent person constantly fears abandonment, being left alone, or the end of the relationship, and every action or behavior is aimed at avoiding this feared outcome.

From a psychological perspective, emotional dependency manifests through several dysfunctional behaviors, including:

- **Obsessive control and jealousy:** The emotionally dependent person has a continuous need to monitor their partner, to know where they are, who they are with, and what they are doing, in an attempt to avoid any situation that might jeopardize the relationship. Jealousy becomes a response to the fear of abandonment and often leads to controlling or manipulative behavior.
- **Submission and personal sacrifice:** To avoid conflict or the possibility of being abandoned, the emotionally dependent person is willing to sacrifice their own desires, needs, and values. They erase themselves for the sake of the partner, placing the other at the center of every decision, even at the cost of their well-being.
- **Fear of loneliness:** Emotional dependency is closely tied to the fear of being alone. The emotionally dependent person prefers to stay in a painful or toxic relationship rather

than face the loneliness and emotional void that would come from breaking up.

- **Continuous search for reassurance:** The emotionally dependent person constantly seeks validation from their partner: they need to feel loved, accepted, and desired, and any sign of detachment, even minimal, is met with great anxiety.
- **Low self-esteem and self-devaluation:** The emotionally dependent person has a highly negative self-image and cannot see their own value except through the eyes of the other. They often live with the idea of not being enough or deserving of love, and they cling to their partner as their only source of confirmation and validation.

In psychodynamic terms, emotional dependency is seen as a regression to infantile stages of emotional development, where the individual has not developed sufficient emotional self-sustainability. In the early years of life, the child depends entirely on caregivers for emotional and physical well-being. If these figures were unable to offer stable, consistent, and unconditional affection, the child may grow up with a sense of emotional insecurity that will be reflected in their adult relationships. The emotionally dependent person, therefore, seeks in their partner the same reassurance and stability they didn't receive as a child, forming relationships characterized by anxious attachment and a constant need for validation.

According to attachment theories, emotional dependency can develop in individuals who experienced insecure attachment styles during childhood, such as "anxious attachment disorder." These individuals tend to approach adult relationships with a constant fear of abandonment, continuously trying to avoid rejection, often at the expense of their emotional well-being. This is accompanied by hyper-protective or hyper-vigilant behavior, making a balanced and healthy relationship impossible.

More broadly, emotional dependency is closely linked to issues of low self-esteem, chronic insecurity, and a lack of self-confidence. The emotionally dependent person does not believe they can find happiness or stability within themselves, so they desperately seek these things externally through their partner.

However, this search is destined to fail, as no relationship, no matter how fulfilling, can fill the inner void that characterizes emotional dependency.

In summary, emotional dependency is a relational pathology: a condition in which the emotional bond, instead of being an experience of mutual growth and freedom, becomes a cage in which the individual loses themselves, their needs, and their identity. From a psychological perspective, healing from emotional dependency involves a personal growth process that includes developing greater self-awareness, rebuilding self-esteem, and learning to live relationships based on reciprocity, respect, and autonomy.

The Difference Between Healthy Love and Emotional Dependency

Healthy love and emotional dependency, although seemingly similar at first glance, are two profoundly different realities. Like the sun and the moon, they share the same sky of relationships but shine with completely different light. While healthy love is a force that nurtures, strengthens, and inspires, emotional dependency is a shadow that silently creeps into the folds of the relationship, making it oppressive, stifling, and often painful. To fully understand this difference, we must delve into the emotional mechanisms, desires, and behaviors that define these two experiences.

Healthy Love: A Dance of Freedom and Sharing

Healthy love is, first and foremost, a choice. It is the meeting of two autonomous individuals, complete in themselves, who decide to walk together, sharing joys, sorrows, and dreams without ever losing sight of their own identity. In healthy love, partners love each other for who they are, not for what the other can offer in terms of reassurance or completion. Each remains themselves, with their own needs, desires, and goals, and this is not perceived as a threat but as a richness.

In a healthy relationship, freedom is a central value. This is not a matter of unrestrained freedom or disinterest, but an emotional space that allows each partner to grow as an individual, to explore their own interests, and to develop their potential, knowing that the other is there, beside them, as support and companion, not as a guardian or controller. Healthy love does not stifle but gives breath. It is like a garden where each flower has its own beauty, its own space to bloom, without one trying to overshadow or take the place of the other.

Another fundamental characteristic of healthy love is reciprocity. In a balanced relationship, both partners give and receive equally. It's not about calculations or exchanges, but a natural flow of emotions, support, and affection that moves in both directions. In a healthy relationship, no one feels neglected or overwhelmed. The needs of both are respected and met, and if problems or conflicts arise, they are addressed with open communication, respect, and understanding. Healthy love is not immune to difficulties but faces challenges as an opportunity to grow together, to deepen the bond without jeopardizing each other's emotional stability.

Finally, healthy love is rooted in trust. Each partner trusts the other, their loyalty, their love, but also their ability to take care of themselves and make decisions that respect the relationship. This trust is not based on constant control but on a sense of mutual security that comes from the awareness of being loved for who one is, not for what one does or gives.

Emotional Dependency: A Bond of Fear and Control

If healthy love is a dance where each partner moves with lightness and respect for the other, emotional dependency is a chain that binds the two partners in a suffocating embrace. In emotional dependency, the other is not seen as a companion to share life with, but as the only source of value, security, and happiness. The dependent individual does not feel complete or enough on their own and therefore places the burden on the other to fill that inner void, to meet emotional needs they cannot satisfy on their own.

In an emotionally dependent relationship, balance is broken. There is no longer freedom, but control. The emotionally dependent person lives in constant fear of losing the other, of being abandoned, and this fear drives obsessive behaviors like extreme jealousy, the need for continuous reassurances, and an exaggerated focus on every small sign of distance or disinterest. Every gesture from the partner is interpreted as a potential threat, and every distance is experienced as a prelude to the end of the relationship.

One of the most evident aspects of emotional dependency is self-erasure. The emotionally dependent person often sacrifices themselves, giving up their own needs, dreams, and desires to conform to what they believe the other wants. There is no longer room for individuality because the sole purpose becomes maintaining the relationship at any cost. In this way, emotional dependency stifles not only one's personal growth but also that of the partner, because love is replaced by need, and need inevitably leads to a form of possession.

Reciprocity, a key characteristic of healthy love, is absent in emotional dependency. The relationship becomes unbalanced: one partner gives much more than they receive, or demands much more than they are willing to offer. There is always an imbalance that translates into frustration, dissatisfaction, and, in the long run, the destruction of the relationship itself. The emotionally dependent person does not give the other space but envelops them in a vortex of demands and expectations that the other, no matter how affectionate, will never be able to fully satisfy.

Another hallmark of emotional dependency is the lack of trust. Unlike healthy love, where trust is a cornerstone, in emotional dependency, trust is always fragile, constantly undermined by doubts and fears. The emotionally dependent person needs to control their partner, to know where they are, what they are doing, who they are with, because they live in constant fear of being betrayed or abandoned. This behavior ends up undermining the relationship itself, generating tensions, conflicts, and growing emotional distance.

Two Visions of Love Compared

In the end, the difference between healthy love and emotional dependency lies in how each individual experiences and perceives themselves and the other. In healthy love, the partner is a traveling companion, a presence that enriches life but does not become indispensable for one's existence. The relationship is a place of growth, freedom, and mutual support. In emotional dependency, however, the other is seen as the only source of value and security, and the relationship becomes a cage in which the emotionally dependent person loses their identity and autonomy.

While healthy love is a conscious choice, renewed every day in freedom and trust, emotional dependency is a compulsive need, an emotional trap that imprisons both partners in a dynamic of fear, control, and insecurity. And like all forms of addiction, emotional dependency can be overcome, but only through a process of self-awareness and personal growth, allowing one to rediscover their value and learn to love in a more authentic and free way.

At its core, healthy love is the meeting of two souls who choose each other, day after day, without chains and without fear, while emotional dependency is the desperate attempt to hold onto someone to avoid facing the loneliness within.

The Confusion Between Romantic Love and the Obsessive Need to Be Loved

There is a fine, almost invisible line that separates romantic love from the obsessive need to be loved. It is a fragile line, often confused and distorted by our emotions, fears, and the expectations that society imposes on us. The desire to be loved, to find a soulmate who completes us, is perhaps one of the deepest needs of the human being. However, when this desire turns into an obsessive need, love loses its purity and beauty, becoming an emotional trap.

Let's imagine for a moment observing a lush garden. Flowers bloom in vibrant colors, and the plants grow strong, nourished by the sunlight and rain. This is romantic love, a love that blooms and grows naturally, where each partner nourishes the other without losing their own roots. But if the gardener starts watering too much, obsessed with the idea that every plant must grow faster and more vigorously, the result will be a waterlogged ground, suffocated by the excess. The flowers will no longer grow but rot. In the same way, the obsessive need to be loved suffocates love, overwhelming it with a flood of expectations and demands that ultimately destroy what was meant to be protected.

In our culture, romantic love is often idealized. We are told stories of great passions, of loves that overcome all obstacles, of soulmates who find each other and, once together, live happily ever after. This myth leads us to believe that true love must be all-consuming, exclusive, that the other must become the center of our existence and the source of all our happiness. Yet, this idealized view of love is dangerous because it confuses love with need. It pushes us to seek in the other not a person with whom to share life, but someone who fills our voids, satisfies our insecurities, and gives us constant validation that we are loved.

This confusion between romantic love and the obsessive need to be loved manifests in various ways. At first, it may seem harmless. Who hasn't wanted to feel loved and special in the eyes of another? But slowly, this desire to be loved can turn into an obsession. You become dependent on the other's words, their gestures, their attention. Love, which should be a free and spontaneous feeling, becomes a constant search for validation. You feel lost, empty, without the other. Every word or gesture becomes a test of love, and if even one small attention is missing, doubt and fear arise that something has changed, that the love is fading.

In this way, the obsessive need to be loved leaves no room for freedom. The other becomes an object, a kind of mirror in which to reflect one's worth. And here lies the great confusion: you no longer love the other for who they are but for how they make you feel. True romantic love is a conscious choice, the desire to share your life with someone without losing yourself. It is a meeting of two complete people who enrich each other. The obsessive need, on the other hand, is the search for an emotional crutch. You don't seek love, you seek certainty, constant confirmation that you are loved, desired, needed.

When trapped in this obsessive need, every small distance, every small sign of the other's independence, is perceived as a betrayal. You become jealous, possessive, and develop a constant fear of abandonment. The relationship stops being a ground for mutual growth and becomes a battlefield, where every day is a struggle for the other's attention and love. But this is not love. Love is not control, it is not possession, it is not the constant demand for reassurance. True love doesn't need chains. The obsessive need, however, chains the other, depriving them of their freedom and suffocating the relationship.

This confusion between love and need often stems from deep insecurity. Those who do not feel enough, who have not developed a solid sense of self-esteem, tend to seek in the other the validation of their worth. Love becomes a way to fill emotional voids. You believe that if the other loves you, then you are worth something, you are important. But this is a dangerous illusion. No one can fill our voids; no one can give us the sense of completeness we seek. Only when we learn to love ourselves, only when we recognize our worth independently of the other's love, can we live a healthy relationship.

True romantic love is freedom. It is knowing that the other loves us but also knowing that, without them, we would still be complete. It is a meeting of two individuals who enrich each other but do not define each other. The obsessive need, on the other hand, is dependency. It is the belief that without the other, we are nothing, that without their approval and love, we are lost.

This confusion between love and need often stems from childhood, from emotional wounds that have never healed. If, as children, we didn't receive the unconditional love we needed, it's likely that as adults, we seek to fill that void through relationships. We look for someone who loves us unconditionally, who never leaves us, who gives us the security we never had. But this search is destined to fail because no love can be so perfect and all-encompassing.

To break this confusion, deep inner work is necessary. We must learn to distinguish between healthy love and the need to be loved. Healthy love is made of freedom, trust, and respect.

The obsessive need, on the other hand, is made of control, fear, and insecurity. Only when we learn to recognize the difference can we begin to live authentic relationships, where love is not a way to fill our voids but a free and reciprocal feeling that enriches both lives.

Ultimately, romantic love is a gift, a meeting of souls who choose each other without chains. The obsessive need to be loved, on the other hand, is an invisible prison, built by fear and insecurity, that prevents us from truly loving and being loved. To experience authentic love, we must first learn to love ourselves, to feel complete without the other, to recognize that our worth does not depend on the love we receive but on the love we know how to give—to ourselves and to others. Only then can we break the confusion between need and love and open ourselves to the true beauty of the romantic bond.

The History of the Concept of Emotional Dependency in Modern Psychology

The concept of emotional dependency, as we know it today, is the result of a long theoretical evolution within modern psychology. It has not always been defined with the clarity and precision we now associate with the term. In fact, the understanding of emotional dependency has undergone a gradual process of definition and exploration, intertwined with the development of disciplines such as psychoanalysis, behavioral psychology, and attachment psychology.

To understand the evolution of the concept, we need to travel back in time to the origins of psychology, when the first pioneers began exploring the complex dynamics of human relationships and love. In the early 20th century, Sigmund Freud, the father of psychoanalysis, introduced the concept of attachment and dependency in his theories on object relations. According to Freud, childhood is the crucial period when the first emotional bonds are formed, and the quality of these early relationships determines the development of personality. For Freud, attachment to the mother or father represented the foundation on which all future relationships are built, and emotional dependency could be seen as a repetition of these early dynamics, in which the adult subject seeks, through relationships, to resolve unresolved conflicts or obtain the love they felt they did not receive as a child.

Freud did not use the term "emotional dependency" as we understand it today, but his writings already hinted at the idea that love and relationships could become a form of psychological dependency. In his early theories, the concept of "dependency" was linked to the notion of "repetition compulsion," in which an individual unconsciously replays the emotional patterns of their childhood in adult relationships, especially those that were unhealthy or traumatic.

In the following years, the understanding of emotional dependency began to take clearer shape through attachment theories, particularly thanks to the work of John Bowlby, one of the leading theorists in child development. In the 1950s, Bowlby developed his attachment theory, studying the bond between children and their primary caregivers. He hypothesized that attachment was a fundamental survival need and that the quality of care received had a profound impact on a child's emotional and relational development. According to Bowlby, secure attachment provided the child with a solid emotional foundation, while insecure attachment, due to neglect, abandonment, or inconsistent care, could lead to emotional and relational difficulties in adulthood.

Bowlby's attachment theory laid the groundwork for understanding emotional dependency as a dysfunctional form of attachment, in which the individual has not developed sufficient internal security and, as a result, constantly seeks in the other the emotional security and stability they have never experienced. Subsequent research conducted by Mary Ainsworth, with her famous "Strange Situation" experiment (1970), deepened the understanding of these attachment styles, outlining secure attachment and the two main insecure attachment styles: anxious-ambivalent and avoidant. It was the anxious-ambivalent attachment that provided one of the first theoretical frameworks for understanding emotional dependency, as in this style, the individual tends to develop an incessant need for reassurance and affection from the other, displaying behaviors of control, possessiveness, and fear of abandonment.

In the 1970s and 1980s, the concept of emotional dependency was enriched by studies in humanistic and behavioral psychology, which began to treat dependency not only as a learned behavior but also as a form of emotional conditioning. Love and affection were seen not only as fundamental needs but also as something that could become distorted, creating pathological dependency similar to substance or other behavioral addictions. Emotional dependency began to be viewed as a condition in which the need to be loved and accepted by the other became so overwhelming that it erased the individual's autonomy.

During this period, transactional analysis, developed by Eric Berne, and existential positional theory helped bring to light the idea that emotional dependency was rooted in dysfunctional and childish relational patterns, where the individual perceives themselves as "not okay" and constantly seeks external confirmation to feel valid. The co-dependency model, developed in the 1980s, further expanded the understanding of emotional dependency by highlighting how it often manifests not only as a one-sided bond but as a reciprocal relational dynamic in which both parties depend on each other in unhealthy ways. Co-dependency, a concept initially linked to the dynamics of families with alcoholics, was also applied to romantic relationships, explaining how partners mutually reinforce each other in a spiral of emotional dependency, seeking validation and reassurance that keep both trapped in a dysfunctional relationship.

In the 1990s and 2000s, emotional dependency was further defined as a true relational pathology. Psychologist and therapist Pia Mellody, one of the leading voices in the field of emotional dependency, wrote foundational books such as *Facing Love Addiction* (1992), in which she described the painful and destructive cycle of relationships based on dependency. Mellody argued that emotional dependency stemmed from low self-esteem and an inability to establish healthy boundaries in relationships. In her view, emotionally dependent people live in a state of constant need and fear, seeking validation from the other and completely losing touch with their autonomous identity.

In the 21st century, the concept of emotional dependency has continued to evolve, becoming increasingly part of the popular and therapeutic psychological debate. Awareness of emotional dependency has grown alongside the increasing focus on mental health and toxic relationships, and today, emotional dependency is recognized as a common problem, though often underestimated. The dynamics of control, possession, and fear of abandonment that characterize emotional dependency have been the subject of numerous studies, highlighting how these dynamics are fueled by individuals' deep insecurities and unrealistic expectations of finding happiness solely in another person.

Conclusion

Today, emotional dependency is considered not only a relational disorder but also an issue that touches on identity and self-esteem. It is a condition that can be overcome through awareness and therapy, but it requires deep inner work. Its history in modern psychology reflects the complex and fascinating journey that has led to a better understanding of the challenges of the human heart, revealing how love, if not properly managed, can turn into an emotional trap that limits personal freedom and mutual growth.

Part 1: Understanding Emotional DependencyChapter 2

The Causes of Emotional Dependency

Emotional dependency does not arise out of nowhere. Like a plant sinking its roots deep into the ground, it sprouts from a combination of psychological, emotional, and environmental factors that shape the individual from childhood. Emotional dependency is not a conscious choice but the result of experiences and conditioning that impact our ability to love and relate to others. It develops over time, like a subtle crack that infiltrates our being, pushing us to seek in others the confirmation of our worth and existence. To truly understand its roots, it is necessary to explore the various levels on which it is built: family, self-esteem, trauma, society, and culture.

1 Roots in Childhood: Attachment and Unconditional Love The first deep cause of emotional dependency lies in early attachment experiences, in the relationship between the child and caregivers, usually the parents. According to John Bowlby's attachment theory, the quality of these early relationships largely determines how we experience relationships as adults. If the child experienced secure attachment, receiving unconditional love, emotional presence, and stability, they will develop an inner sense of security that will accompany them into future relationships. However, when attachment was insecure—due to emotionally absent, unstable, critical, or unpredictable parents—the child grows up feeling that they must earn love, constantly striving for others' attention and approval.

The child who did not receive the love they needed will develop a deep wound, a sense of emptiness that will carry into adulthood. This emptiness becomes the ground in which emotional dependency grows, as the individual seeks in others what they never had: love, security, confirmation of their worth. In essence, emotional dependency stems from an insatiable need to be loved, to be seen and accepted for who they are, a need rooted in deficient or dysfunctional emotional experiences from early childhood.

2 Fragile Self-Esteem: The Heart of Dependency Another key factor in the development of emotional dependency is low self-esteem. Those who suffer from emotional dependency often do not believe they are worthy enough. They live with the constant feeling of being inadequate, of not deserving love, and therefore cling desperately to anyone who gives them attention or affection. Fragile self-esteem is like unstable ground on which it is impossible to build a solid emotional foundation; as a result, the individual seeks their identity and worth outside themselves, relying entirely on others' judgment and affection.

Low self-esteem often develops from critical or devaluing experiences, possibly related to hypercritical, absent, or emotionally unstable parents. Growing up in an environment where love is conditional—where affection is given only in exchange for specific behaviors or achievements—leads to internalizing the idea that one's worth is tied to actions, not being. This results in relationships where the person constantly seeks validation of their worth through their partner's approval, becoming unable to find this validation within themselves.

3 **Fear of Abandonment and Emotional Emptiness** Fear of abandonment is one of the main drivers of emotional dependency. Those who suffer from it live with the constant fear of being left alone, abandoned by the ones they love. This fear has deep roots, often tied to abandonment or loss experiences in childhood. Sometimes these are real events, such as parental separation, the loss of a significant figure, or the feeling of being neglected during emotionally critical moments. Other times, the fear of abandonment arises from subtler experiences, such as the lack of consistent emotional attention from parents.

This fear of being abandoned leads the emotionally dependent person to develop anxious attachment, where even the slightest sign of detachment from the other is experienced as an existential threat. The dependent individual clings to their partner, fearing that if the other person distances themselves, they will be forced to confront an emotional void they cannot face alone. As a result, their relationships are often characterized by jealousy, possessiveness, and control, as the dependent person desperately tries to avoid the end of the relationship.

4 **Emotional Trauma and Scars of the Soul** Another crucial element contributing to emotional dependency is emotional trauma. Painful experiences in childhood or adolescence, such as physical, emotional, or sexual abuse, can leave deep scars that affect how the individual relates to others. These traumas create an emotional wound that often goes unrecognized or unaddressed and manifests in adulthood through a constant search for love and reassurance.

Trauma can create a distorted perception of love: those who have experienced violence or neglect may develop a tendency to confuse pain with affection, unconsciously seeking relationships where pain and sacrifice are considered proof of love. In these cases, emotional dependency becomes a form of compensation for the trauma experienced, an endless search for a savior figure who can finally fill the void of love and security.

5 Cultural and Social Pressures: Love as an Unrealistic Ideal

The society and culture we live in play a fundamental role in the construction of emotional dependency. Our culture has built a myth of romantic love, an unrealistic ideal in which love is seen as the solution to all problems, the pinnacle of a happy life. Movies, songs, and novels constantly present the image of two people meeting and finding complete fulfillment in their relationship. This myth, however appealing, creates unrealistic expectations, pushing us to believe that only through another person can we feel complete and happy.

This social pressure can fuel emotional dependency, leading us to believe that being single or alone is a condition of failure or incompleteness. Love is idealized and sanctified, and consequently, we end up seeking it at all costs, even at the expense of our well-being. In this way, emotional dependency feeds off the need to conform to a cultural model in which being loved by another becomes synonymous with success and personal fulfillment.

6 Familial Conditioning and Learned Relationship Models

Finally, another crucial factor in the development of emotional dependency is familial conditioning. Often, without realizing it, we replicate in our adult relationships the relational models we learned in childhood. If we grew up in a family where love was conditional, where relationships were based on control, manipulation, or emotional abuse, we are likely to replicate these dynamics in our romantic relationships. From an early age, we learn that love is something that must be earned, that it is unstable and unpredictable, and we carry this belief into our adult lives.

Dysfunctional family dynamics, such as overprotection, emotional manipulation, or lack of healthy boundaries, can predispose us to emotional dependency by teaching us to sacrifice ourselves to maintain the bond with others. This leads to relationships based on need, fear of loneliness, and a constant search for approval.

ConclusionEmotional dependency is a complex interplay of emotional, psychological, and social factors that develop over time, rooted in childhood experiences and unresolved emotional wounds. It is not simply an inability to love in a healthy way but a deep and visceral need to be loved and accepted to fill an inner void. However, understanding the causes of emotional dependency is the first step toward healing. Only by acknowledging our wounds, confronting our past, and learning to love ourselves for who we are can we break the cycle of dependency and build healthy relationships based on authentic love and freedom.

Psychological Factors: Low Self-Esteem, Fear of Abandonment

Emotional dependency is like a mosaic made up of delicate and often painful fragments, pieced together to form a complex picture. Two of the most important components of this picture are low self-esteem and the fear of abandonment. These two psychological elements work together, feeding off each other, to create an inner dynamic that drives a person to desperately seek in others the validation of their worth and emotional security that they cannot find within themselves. They are invisible but powerful forces that shape how we relate, love, and seek to be loved.

Low Self-Esteem: A Void That Demands to Be Filled

Imagine self-esteem as the foundation of a house. If the foundation is solid, the house can withstand the winds and storms of life. But if it is fragile, every small tremor can shake the structure, causing cracks that widen over time. Those who suffer from emotional dependency often live with these fragile foundations, invisible cracks that silently extend deep into their identity. Low self-esteem is one of the main roots of emotional dependency, and it is a problem that arises long before a person enters into a relationship.

Low self-esteem is a deeply ingrained belief of not being good enough, of being unworthy of love, or lacking intrinsic value. It is an inner voice that constantly whispers doubts: "You're not good enough. You don't deserve love. No one will really love you unless you do more." This voice becomes a constant companion, carving a sense of inadequacy in the heart of those who suffer from it. The person begins to seek in others a continuous confirmation, a reassurance that can temporarily soothe that feeling of inner emptiness. Every time the partner shows affection or appreciation, the person feels momentarily relieved, as if those words could fill the void left by fragile self-esteem.

But this relief is fleeting. Like a leaky bucket that can never hold water, the need for validation returns quickly, stronger than before. The person becomes dependent on the attention and love of others to feel worthy. They do not love themselves for who they are, but only for how they are perceived by others. Their self-esteem becomes a sort of distorted mirror, reflecting only the value that others attribute to them, and if that mirror cracks—if the partner distances themselves even for a moment—the person immediately feels lost, devoid of a positive self-image.

Those who suffer from low self-esteem in emotional dependency often make compromises that cause them pain. They sacrifice themselves, put their needs aside, give up their dreams, just to maintain the relationship. They convince themselves that if they do everything their partner wants, maybe they will be loved. This behavior is nothing more than an attempt to earn love because, in their mind, love is something that must be deserved, not something that is freely given. Love becomes a sort of emotional contract where every gesture must be balanced by a confirmation of value, and the relationship turns into a continuous negotiation between giving and receiving attention to fill the inner void.

Fear of Abandonment: An Abyss That Threatens to Devour Us

Alongside low self-esteem, the fear of abandonment is the other dark force that fuels emotional dependency. It is an ancient, primordial fear rooted in the deepest experiences of childhood. In those early years of life, the child is completely dependent on caregivers for their physical and emotional survival. If those bonds are marked by instability, lack of affection, or abandonment, the child grows up with a wound that accompanies them for life.

This wound manifests in adulthood as a constant fear of being left alone, of being abandoned, of not being enough to hold on to those we love. The person who suffers from emotional dependency lives with the anguish of losing their partner, and this fear becomes an overwhelming presence, influencing every aspect of the relationship. Every small gesture or word from the partner is interpreted through the lens of this fear: an unanswered message, a distracted look, an evening spent apart become signs that love is ending, that abandonment is imminent.

The fear of abandonment pushes the person to obsessively control their partner, constantly seeking reassurance of love and presence. They become jealous, possessive, living with the anxiety of always knowing where the other person is, with whom, and what they are thinking. Even emotional distance is experienced as a wound, and the relationship becomes a constant struggle to keep the other person close. This fear creates a suffocating energy in the relationship, where the other feels constantly under pressure, as if they must always prove their love to avoid hurting their partner.

But the cruel irony of the fear of abandonment is that the more one tries to hold on to the other, the more they risk deteriorating the relationship. The emotionally dependent person, in an attempt to prevent abandonment, ends up creating a stifling dynamic that wears down the partner, paradoxically pushing them to seek freedom and distance. This only confirms the dependent person's fear, who then enters a vicious cycle: the greater the fear of abandonment, the more they try to control the other; the more they try to control the other, the more the relationship breaks down.

The Interaction Between Low Self-Esteem and Fear of Abandonment

Low self-esteem and fear of abandonment intertwine in a vicious cycle that fuels emotional dependency. The person with low self-esteem does not feel worthy enough and seeks validation from others. However, the fear of abandonment, always lurking in the background, makes it impossible to live the relationship serenely. Every sign of distancing is perceived as a threat to their identity, as tangible proof of their inadequacy.

This creates a relational dynamic in which the dependent individual becomes incapable of experiencing a healthy, balanced love. They cling desperately to their partner, asking for more and more reassurance, validation, and love. But love experienced in this way is no longer love: it is need. It is the fear of being alone, the belief that without the other, one is destined to disappear, to lose their identity. And at this crucial point, the line between love and dependency blurs.

People who live with low self-esteem and the fear of abandonment cannot see themselves as worthy of love regardless of the circumstances. Every act of affection is experienced as a saving gesture, an anchor to cling to in order not to be swallowed by the void. But this anchoring to the other only perpetuates suffering because no partner, no matter how loving, can fill the void left by a lack of self-esteem.

Conclusion

Low self-esteem and fear of abandonment are two forces that, together, form the foundation of emotional dependency. They are like two shadows that follow the individual in their relationships, making them incapable of living love with peace and freedom. For those who suffer from emotional dependency, the other becomes a sort of emotional anchor, a refuge from a sense of emptiness and inadequacy that cannot be filled alone.

However, recognizing these dynamics is the first step toward healing. Only by addressing low self-esteem, learning to see one's own worth independently of the other, and working on the fear of abandonment can one break the cycle of emotional dependency. Authentic love can only be born when we are able to love ourselves without fear, without obsessive need, and without depending on the other to confirm our worth.

Cultural and Social Factors: Models of Love in the Media and Families

Emotional dependency is not formed solely within the mind and heart of an individual; it is also shaped by the broader influences of society and the culture that surrounds us. In a world where love is often portrayed in an idealized, dramatic, or possessive manner, it is not surprising that many of us develop unrealistic expectations and dysfunctional behaviors in relationships. The models of love presented to us by the media and within our families act as invisible but powerful forces, contributing to a distorted idea of love that fuels emotional dependency.

Idealized Love in the Media: The Myth of the "Happy Ending"

Modern media, particularly cinema, television, and social media, play a crucial role in shaping our ideas about love. From childhood, we are exposed to stories that tell us that true love is the cornerstone of a happy and complete life. From classic fairy tales to Hollywood romances, love is often depicted as a powerful force capable of overcoming any obstacle. In common narratives, love is the ultimate goal, the moment when two people, after countless challenges and struggles, finally find each other and live "happily ever after." This image, though captivating and attractive, feeds the idea that love is something extraordinary and all-encompassing, capable of solving all problems and bringing a sense of absolute completeness.

However, this vision of love is unrealistic and potentially dangerous. The myth of the happy ending does not account for the complexity of real relationships, which are made of ups and downs, compromises, and, at times, failures. When we are constantly shown that love is a perfect experience and that true love must be overwhelming and passionate, we begin to believe that any relationship that does not meet these ideal standards is flawed or incomplete. This can lead people to seek in others a level of perfection and romance that does not exist in real life.

Media representations of love often promote the notion of a partner who "completes us." This idea, made famous by films like *Jerry Maguire* with the iconic line "You complete me," suggests that without another person, we are fundamentally incomplete. This message is deeply rooted in romantic culture and creates immense pressure. Those living in a context that promotes this vision of love may feel driven to desperately search for a partner to fill that inner void, which, instead, should be filled through personal growth and self-esteem.

The music industry, with its poignant and passionate songs, often further fuels this distorted vision. Many love songs speak of suffering, extreme sacrifices, and a love so powerful that it obliterates all other aspects of life. This extreme romantic model creates a link between the concept of love and that of pain and obsession, as if to love inevitably means sacrificing oneself, one's dreams, and one's freedom in the name of a romantic ideal that exists only in stories.

Social Media and Perfect Love: The Illusion of Relationship Happiness

In recent decades, with the rise of social media, this phenomenon has worsened further. Platforms like Instagram, Facebook, and TikTok have become showcases where people display the most polished and idealized versions of their relationships. We see seemingly perfect couples, always smiling, always in love, living dream lives. Pictures of romantic vacations, elegant dinners, and affectionate gestures paint a distorted reality in which love appears to be always joyful, free from conflict, and without shadows.

This constant exposure to models of perfect love creates unsustainable cultural pressure. Many people, unconsciously, begin comparing their own love lives with what they see on social media, forgetting that what is shown is only a partial, if not completely fictional, representation. This constant comparison leads to feelings of dissatisfaction, inadequacy, and the belief that if one's relationship does not meet these standards of perfection, then something is wrong. The result is increased insecurity, which can contribute to developing emotional dependency, where one seeks in the other the security and perfection reflected on screens but unattainable in real life.

Family Models: Love as a Learned Dynamic

While the media create models of idealized and perfect love, the family of origin plays an equally crucial role in shaping our relational expectations. The way we experienced and observed love relationships during childhood deeply influences how we live and perceive love as adults. From an early age, we learn from the family environment how affection, love, and care are expressed. If we grew up in a family with dysfunctional dynamics—characterized by conflicts, emotional manipulation, or abuse—it is very likely that we replicate these patterns in our adult relationships.

In many families, love is presented as conditional. Perhaps we were loved only when we got good grades, behaved well, or met our parents' expectations. This creates a distorted view of love, where we learn to believe that affection must be earned, that love is never unconditional but always tied to performance or behavior. As adults, this can manifest as a compulsive need to please others, to sacrifice oneself to receive love, since we unconsciously believe that love must be deserved.

In families where one or both parents were emotionally absent, a fear of abandonment may develop, driving an obsessive need for the other person's presence to avoid reliving that sense of loneliness experienced in childhood. Similarly, if we grew up in a family where one parent was excessively possessive or controlling, we might replicate these dynamics, seeking to control our partner or be controlled in order to feel secure.

Families are also the first sources of lessons on how to handle conflict. If we grew up in an environment where conflicts were avoided or repressed, we may struggle to address issues in our relationships, accumulating frustration and fostering a dynamic of emotional dependency where we fear confrontation out of fear of losing the other. Conversely, if family conflicts were excessive and destructive, we might develop a distorted view of relationships, believing that love must always be tumultuous and filled with drama.

The Culture of Sacrifice and Possessive Love

Another important cultural factor that contributes to emotional dependency is the idea of love as total self-sacrifice. In the cultural tradition of many countries, and especially in patriarchal contexts, love is often associated with sacrifice, particularly for women. Traditional cultural narratives, passed down through generations, have often celebrated figures of lovers or spouses who completely sacrifice themselves for the other, who renounce their own desires and aspirations to fully dedicate themselves to the relationship. This model of love-sacrifice creates cultural pressure that leads people to believe that loving means always and inevitably putting the other person first, even at the cost of losing oneself.

Similarly, the culture of possessive love—where love is seen as an exclusive and absolute right over the other—can reinforce emotional dependency. Jealousy and control, which should be warning signs in relationships, are sometimes interpreted as proofs of passionate love. Popular culture often romanticizes the idea that a jealous or possessive partner acts that way because they love too much, reinforcing the notion that healthy love must be imbued with fear of loss and obsessive attachment.

Conclusion

Cultural and social factors play a profound role in shaping our expectations and beliefs about love. From the idealized models presented by the media to the dynamics learned within families, we are constantly exposed to narratives that influence how we experience relationships. When these narratives promote an unrealistic, possessive, or conditional vision of love, they can help lay the foundation for emotional dependency, pushing us to seek in others what we should first find in ourselves: security, self-esteem, and unconditional love. Only through awareness of these cultural and social influences can we begin to free ourselves from them and build healthier, more authentic relationships, based on freedom and mutual respect.

Influence of Childhood: Relationships with Parents and Attachment Figures

Childhood is the secret and profound place where the seeds of our future relationships are planted. It is during these formative years that we learn what it means to love and be loved, to nurture and be nurtured. Relationships with parents and attachment figures play a crucial role in shaping our inner world, defining how we emotionally connect with others, and particularly how we perceive ourselves within a relationship. These primary bonds not only influence our vision of love, but also determine our ability to develop emotional security or, conversely, to suffer from emotional dependency.

The Power of Attachment: The First Lessons of Love

When we come into the world, we are vulnerable creatures, completely dependent on those who care for us. We cannot yet speak, we do not understand the world around us, but one thing is certain: we need love. Attachment figures—usually parents, but they can also be grandparents, aunts, uncles, or other adults who play a crucial role in our growth—are our first teachers of love. Through their gestures of care, protection, and affection, we begin to build a picture of what an emotional relationship is.

According to attachment theory developed by John Bowlby, early attachment experiences create a mental model that accompanies us throughout life, influencing how we relate to others as adults. If parents or attachment figures respond to our needs with love, attention, and consistency, we learn that the world is a safe place, that we are loved for who we are, and that we can trust others. This type of attachment, called secure attachment, lays the foundation for a healthy and independent relational life. The individual develops the ability to experience love as a place of growth and freedom, where affection can be given and received without fear.

But when these attachment figures do not respond to the child's needs consistently or adequately, when the bond is marked by instability, emotional absence, or even abuse, the individual's emotional foundation is cracked. Here, emotional dependency is born as a response to the void left by the love that was not given in the necessary measure.

Insecure Attachment: The Roots of Emotional Dependency

A child who does not receive consistent emotional care or who grows up in an unstable family environment develops insecure attachment, a condition that manifests itself in two main forms: anxious-ambivalent attachment and avoidant attachment. These models of insecure attachment are at the root of many dynamics of emotional dependency, as they teach the child to experience relationships as a source of anxiety, fear, and confusion.

- **Anxious-Ambivalent Attachment**: In this attachment style, the child lives in a state of constant uncertainty. The attachment figures are intermittently present—sometimes they respond to the child's needs, other times they are absent or emotionally distant. This leads the child to develop a constant fear of abandonment. This uncertainty fuels emotional dependency: the child learns that love is unstable, unpredictable, and that to receive it, they must be constantly vigilant and ready to seek reassurance. This model is reproduced later in adult relationships, where the individual desperately seeks approval and affection from their partner, fearing that any sign of detachment may foreshadow abandonment.

- **Avoidant Attachment**: In other situations, parents or attachment figures are emotionally unavailable or rejecting. To protect themselves from the pain of continuous rejection, the child learns not to trust others and to suppress their own emotional needs. However, this apparent emotional independence is only a facade. As an adult, the individual with avoidant attachment may seem detached, but in reality, they are prisoners of a deep fear of intimacy and an equally strong desire for connection. Emotional dependency can manifest in this case as an unconscious search for someone who can fill the emotional void created by the lack of love in early childhood.

In both cases, childhood leaves an emotional wound that shapes how the individual experiences and perceives love in adult relationships. This wound creates a constant feeling of inadequacy, of not being worthy of love, and of having to do everything to earn the other's affection. The result is a relationship where love turns into obsessive need, and the partner becomes a kind of emotional anchor, the only source of security and stability.

The Lack of Unconditional Love: The Root of Emotional Emptiness

A fundamental aspect that determines emotional dependency is the lack of unconditional love during childhood. Unconditional love is the kind of love a child should receive simply for existing, without having to do anything to earn it. However, not all parents are able to offer this type of love. Some are too absorbed in their own emotional problems, economic difficulties, or past wounds and are unable to give the child the affection and attention they need.

When the child perceives that love is conditional—that they must be good, do their duty, or meet expectations to be loved—they develop a distorted idea of love. They grow up with the belief that affection must be earned, and as an adult, they reproduce this dynamic in romantic relationships. This results in emotional dependency, where the person constantly tries to please the partner, sacrificing themselves to maintain the relationship, believing they are not worthy of love for who they are, but only for what they do.

Emotionally Absent Parents: Loneliness and Fear of Abandonment

Another factor contributing to emotional dependency is the presence of emotionally absent parents. Even though they may be physically present, some parents are unable to respond to the child's emotional needs. Perhaps due to their own wounds, difficulties in the relationship, or personal issues, they are unable to provide the warmth, presence, and affection the child needs to feel secure. This emotional absence leaves the child with a deep sense of loneliness, which they carry into adulthood, where it manifests as a constant fear of abandonment.

The fear of abandonment becomes a constant companion in adult relationships. Those who have experienced emotionally deprived relationships with their parents tend to desperately seek connection in romantic relationships, fearing that if the other person leaves, even momentarily, they will be left alone, as they were in childhood. This fear fuels emotional dependency, pushing the individual to control the partner, seek continuous reassurance, and live in anxiety about being abandoned.

Parental Models and Family Conditioning

Finally, family dynamics themselves—beyond the direct relationship with parents—profoundly influence the formation of emotional dependency. If we grow up in a family where parents have dysfunctional relationships, we tend to replicate those patterns. If a child observes that their father or mother is completely emotionally dependent on the other or that one of the parents constantly sacrifices themselves to maintain the relationship, they will unconsciously learn that love requires sacrifice, self-annihilation, or control.

The relational models we observe as children become part of our unconscious, and without realizing it, we bring them into our adult relationships. If the child sees that love is unstable or marked by conflict, they may grow up believing that all relationships are like this and accept dependency dynamics as normal, without ever questioning their need to find stability and security in the other.

Conclusion

Relationships with parents and attachment figures during childhood lay the foundation for our emotional world. If these relationships are marked by unconditional love, attention, and stability, we grow up with the ability to experience healthy relationships based on trust and reciprocity. But when these relationships are lacking, unstable, or marked by absence, we learn to seek in others the emotional security we never received. Emotional dependency is, therefore, a response to a deep wound: the unresolved need for love and security that drives us to seek in others what we cannot find within ourselves. Only by addressing these wounds and recognizing the patterns we have learned can we begin a path to healing and build healthier, more liberated relationships.

Emotional Wounds: Trauma and Lack of Affection

Emotional wounds are invisible scars we carry within us, etched in the deepest part of our being. These wounds do not bleed like physical ones, but their pain is just as real and persistent. They manifest through our behaviors, in the relationships we build, and often in our inability to love in a healthy way. Trauma and lack of affection during childhood are the main causes of these emotional wounds, and they manifest in adult life as emotional dependency, anxiety, fear of abandonment, and a constant search for validation from others.

Lack of Affection: A Void That Cannot Be Filled

Affection is the emotional nourishment every child needs to grow and develop in a healthy way. Without this nourishment, a void is created, an inner abyss that accompanies the individual throughout their life. Lack of affection is one of the deepest and most difficult emotional wounds to heal, as it touches the primary need to feel loved and accepted for who we are. A child who does not receive love, attention, and warmth from their parents or caregivers develops a constant sense of inadequacy and insecurity. They unconsciously convince themselves that if they were not loved by those who were supposed to love them unconditionally, then there must be something wrong with them.

This belief takes root deeply and grows over time, transforming into a perception of self characterized by low self-esteem and chronic insecurity. A child who has not received the necessary affection often develops emotional dependency in adulthood, constantly seeking to fill that relational void with the love of a partner or other people. The idea of not being enough becomes a constant torment, a shadow that accompanies every relationship. Every gesture of love, every affectionate word becomes a drug they cannot do without, because for a heart starved of love, even the smallest attention can seem essential for survival.

But the truth is that no external love can truly fill the emotional void created by the lack of primary affection. The person suffering from emotional dependency enters relationships with the hope of finding in them the completeness they have never experienced. However, every time the partner moves away, even temporarily, that void resurfaces with force, bringing with it fear, anxiety, and a deep sense of inadequacy. The partner becomes not so much a person to love but a kind of emotional anchor, the only source of security and stability, and the bond turns into a form of dependency that stifles the relationship itself.

Emotional Trauma: Deep Wounds That Shape the Soul

Emotional traumas, especially those experienced during childhood, leave even deeper and more complex scars. While lack of affection can create a feeling of emptiness and loneliness, traumas—such as abandonment, physical or emotional abuse, domestic violence, or the loss of an attachment figure—leave an indelible mark on the psyche. Trauma is not just a moment of pain; it is an event that fractures identity, leaving the child—and later the adult—with a perpetual sense of danger and insecurity. It is like living constantly on the edge, as if the world could collapse at any moment.

When a child experiences trauma, an emotional fracture occurs. Trust in the world and the people around them is broken. If a parent, the figure who should provide protection and unconditional love, becomes the source of pain or abuse, the child not only loses the security of being loved but also internalizes a sense of guilt and shame. Often, the traumatized child convinces themselves that they are somehow responsible for the pain they have suffered, and this belief crystallizes into an emotional wound they carry with them throughout their life.

In adulthood, these wounds manifest in different ways. One of the most common forms is emotional dependency, where the person desperately seeks someone who can repair the emotional damage they have suffered. The individual who has experienced childhood trauma often develops anxious attachment, characterized by a constant fear of abandonment and an incessant need for reassurance. Love becomes a refuge from a world that seems hostile and dangerous, but at the same time, the trauma makes it difficult to fully trust the other person, creating a complex dynamic of desire and fear.

A person who has experienced emotional trauma may develop a disorganized attachment behavior, oscillating between a desperate need for love and an inability to accept it fully out of fear of being hurt again. This creates a painful dance in relationships, where the individual intensely desires intimacy but withdraws every time vulnerability becomes too strong. This ambivalence leads to emotional dependency, where the relationship becomes both a source of comfort and anguish, a spiral of conflicting emotions that slowly erodes the soul.

The Impact of Emotional Wounds in Adult Relationships

When these emotional wounds are not recognized and healed, they manifest in every adult relationship, particularly in romantic relationships. The person who has experienced trauma or lived without affection approaches love with the unconscious belief that it can solve everything, that it can finally repair what was broken. But this belief is the fertile ground on which emotional dependency is born. Love is not experienced as a conscious and free choice but as a necessity, an insatiable need that, if not met, reawakens the primary pain of unhealed wounds.

Emotional wounds push the person to seek constant validation from the partner, as the fear of abandonment is always present. Every gesture, every word from the partner is analyzed, weighed, searching for signs that confirm or deny their affection. The result is a stifling dynamic in which the partner unknowingly becomes responsible for maintaining the fragile emotional balance of the other. But no one can bear the weight of another's wounds forever. Thus, the relationship, which was born with the expectation of bringing healing, becomes a trap for both, an emotional prison that prevents them from growing.

The Path to Healing Emotional Wounds

Emotional wounds, whether caused by trauma or lack of affection, do not disappear on their own. They are like fractures that, if not treated, can only worsen over time. However, the good news is that these wounds can be healed if recognized and addressed with awareness. The first step towards healing is recognizing that they exist, that the pain we feel in our relationships is not caused solely by the partner or current circumstances, but has its roots in past events that were never fully processed.

Therapy can be a powerful means of addressing these traumas. Through psychotherapy, particularly approaches like attachment therapy or trauma therapy, it is possible to explore the roots of one's pain and begin to heal. Learning to rebuild self-esteem, cultivate a sense of inner security, and understand that love cannot be used as a medicine to heal past wounds, but must be experienced as a reciprocal and conscious choice, is fundamental to freeing oneself from emotional dependency.

Conclusion

The emotional wounds created by trauma and lack of affection during childhood are invisible scars that profoundly shape how we love and are loved. These wounds are not seen, but they are felt in every relationship, especially in romantic relationships. They drive the individual to desperately seek in others what they never received: love, acceptance, and security. However, the path to healing is possible. Only by facing these wounds and learning to recognize them for what they are can we begin to free ourselves from the cycle of emotional dependency and live love not as a need but as a free and reciprocal choice, based on true self-knowledge and acceptance.

Part 1: Understanding Emotional DependencyChapter 3

The Dynamics of Dependency in Relationships

Relationships are delicate weavings of emotions, needs, and desires, where two people meet and try to walk together.

However, when emotional dependency creeps into a relationship, the bond that should be a source of growth and exchange turns into an emotional trap, where love becomes intertwined with control, fear, and self-loss. The dynamics of emotional dependency in relationships are subtle yet powerful, and they can slowly erode the very essence of the bond, drawing both partners into a vortex of anxiety, obsession, and need.

The Vicious Cycle of Need and Reassurance

At the core of emotional dependency is a vicious cycle revolving around the need for reassurance. The emotionally dependent person constantly lives with the fear of being abandoned, of not being enough, of not being loved. This fear drives them to continuously seek confirmation and reassurance from their partner through affectionate gestures, words, or even just their constant presence. Every moment of emotional or physical distance is experienced with anxiety, as if it were a warning sign that something might go wrong, that love might slip away.

The need for reassurance becomes a sort of invisible addiction. The dependent person cannot help but seek constant validation of their worth and the emotional bond from the other. But, as with all addictions, this one is destined never to be fully satisfied. Every reassurance provides only temporary relief, a fleeting pause from the anguish, but soon the fear returns, stronger than before. And so, the search for confirmation becomes incessant, feeding a cycle that repeats endlessly.

The partner, for their part, may progressively feel overwhelmed by these demands. Initially, they may respond with love and patience, trying to ease the other's anxieties. But over time, this dynamic becomes suffocating. The partner begins to perceive that nothing they do is ever enough, that every action is interpreted as either a proof of love or, conversely, a threat to the relationship. This leads to a growing rift because the continuous need for reassurance from the emotionally dependent person creates an atmosphere of tension and emotional stress.

Control Disguised as Love

Another characteristic element of emotional dependency dynamics in relationships is control. The emotionally dependent person, driven by the fear of being abandoned, tends to want to control every aspect of the relationship and their partner. This control is not experienced as intentional manipulation but is often interpreted as a form of "care" or "concern" for the other. They want to know where their partner is, who they are with, what they are doing, and every distance, whether emotional or physical, is perceived as a threatening sign.

Control in emotionally dependent relationships is not always explicit. It doesn't necessarily manifest through direct demands or impositions but through a more subtle form of emotional control. The dependent person may display constant jealousy and insecurity, causing the partner to feel guilty whenever they distance themselves, even briefly. This dynamic creates an environment where the partner feels constantly pressured, as if they must continuously prove their love to quell the other's insecurities.

However, control never brings the emotional security that is hoped for. On the contrary, it ends up pushing the partner away, who feels trapped in a web of expectations and emotional demands. The result is that the more the emotionally dependent person tries to hold onto the partner, the more they drive them toward escape. This, in turn, intensifies the fear of abandonment, further fueling the cycle of control and dependency.

Self-Annulment: When Love Becomes Sacrifice

One of the most painful aspects of emotional dependency dynamics is self-annulment. The dependent person is willing to do anything to maintain the relationship, even at the cost of sacrificing their own needs, desires, and values. This happens because, deep down, the emotionally dependent person doesn't feel worthy of love simply for who they are. They believe that to be loved, they must do something, give more than they receive, always be available, understanding, and ready to set themselves aside for the other.

This sacrifice can take many forms: giving up their own dreams, avoiding conflicts out of fear of losing the partner, accepting unacceptable behaviors, or living constantly to please the other. The emotionally dependent person fears that if they assert their own needs or express dissent, they will be abandoned. And so, day after day, they set aside a part of themselves, gradually becoming a faded version of the person they once were.

But this self-annulment never leads to happiness or security in the relationship. On the contrary, the more a person sacrifices, the more frustration and emptiness grow. Love, which should be a source of mutual nourishment, becomes a trap where one's identity is lost. In their attempt to maintain the relationship, the emotionally dependent person ends up living an inauthentic life, where their true emotions and aspirations are repressed.

The "Savior" Partner: The Need to Be Saved

In emotionally dependent relationships, the partner is often seen as a sort of savior. The emotionally dependent person enters the relationship with the unconscious hope that the other can heal their emotional wounds, fill their voids, and give them the sense of completeness they have never experienced on their own. The partner thus becomes an almost mythic figure, the sole source of happiness and security.

This dynamic creates immense pressure on the partner, who finds themselves cast in an impossible role. No person, no matter how loving or present, can truly save another. Love can be a healing force, but it cannot solve deep-rooted issues of self-esteem and emotional wounds. Consequently, the partner of the emotionally dependent individual starts to feel overwhelmed by the expectations, knowing that they can never fully meet the other's emotional needs.

The problem, however, is that the emotionally dependent person cannot see the other for who they truly are: a human being with their own fragilities and limits. Instead, they project onto them the image of a savior, an emotional anchor, and when this image inevitably cracks, deep frustration and disappointment set in. This further fuels the cycle of dependency because, instead of addressing their own internal wounds, the emotionally dependent person desperately tries to make the relationship work as if it alone could provide an escape from the pain.

Co-Dependency: A Dance of Mutual Needs

In many emotionally dependent relationships, it is not just one person who is dependent. Often, a co-dependency dynamic is created, in which both partners emotionally depend on each other, but in different ways. One partner may be the "needy" one, while the other takes on the role of the "savior," creating a kind of dance where each tries to fulfill the other's needs, without ever fully succeeding.

Co-dependency is a dynamic in which both people are trapped in a cycle of mutual need. The partner who tries to "save" the other may feel necessary, indispensable, while the emotionally dependent individual clings to the role of the needy one. This creates a symbiotic relationship where both partners emotionally feed off each other but, at the same time, imprison one another. Neither can truly grow or be free because they both need the other to feel complete.

Conclusion

The dynamics of emotional dependency in relationships are complex and subtle, woven into a cycle of need, fear, and control that can slowly erode the emotional health of both partners. The constant search for reassurance, emotional control, self-annulment, and co-dependency are all manifestations of a bond that, instead of nourishing, drains.

But there is a way out. Awareness of these dynamics is the first step toward healing. Only by recognizing dependency and confronting one's emotional wounds can the cycle be broken and healthier relationships built, based on mutual love, freedom, and respect. Truly loving does not mean possessing or depending on the other, but walking together as two complete individuals, capable of sharing without losing themselves.

Key Characteristics of an Emotionally Dependent Relationship

Emotionally dependent relationships are intense but often distorted emotional entanglements. They arise from the illusion that love is a primary need, a kind of emotional anchor without which we cannot survive. In this type of bond, love is not experienced as a free and mutual feeling but rather as an act of emotional compensation, where one or both partners try to fill deep voids and heal wounds that have never healed. Emotionally dependent relationships are characterized by a dynamic in which fear, control, and self-annulment replace trust, freedom, and mutual growth.

1. The Constant Fear of Abandonment

One of the most distinctive elements of an emotionally dependent relationship is the persistent fear of being abandoned. This fear, often rooted in childhood traumas or deep insecurities, accompanies every moment of the relationship. The dependent person lives with constant anxiety that the partner might distance themselves, that love might fade, and that their life could collapse into the void of abandonment. Every small sign of distance, even a simple silence or a misinterpreted gesture, can trigger a wave of anxiety and obsessive behaviors aimed at reassuring themselves that the relationship is still stable.

This fear manifests in various ways: continuous requests for confirmation, the need to hear "I love you" repeated over and over, and a relentless search for proof that the partner hasn't changed their mind. The relationship becomes a sort of battle against uncertainty, where the emotionally dependent person tries to ward off abandonment by seeking constant closeness and control over the partner. However, this dynamic only feeds the same fear because the more the partner feels suffocated by emotional demands, the more they distance themselves, creating a vicious cycle of insecurity and anxiety.

2. Control and Obsessive Jealousy

Control is another dominant characteristic of emotionally dependent relationships. The dependent person, terrified of losing the other, seeks to keep the partner under constant supervision. This need for control is not always conscious and can take subtle forms, such as the need to always know where the other is, who they are with, what they are doing, or more explicit forms like obsessive jealousy. Even innocent gestures, like a conversation with a friend or a delayed response to a message, can be interpreted as signs of disinterest or, worse, betrayal.

Jealousy becomes a constant in these relationships. Every interaction the partner has with the outside world is seen as a threat, a potential danger to the stability of the relationship. The partner is no longer perceived as an autonomous individual with their own life and freedom but as a kind of emotional property, to be controlled and guarded. Control becomes a defense mechanism, a way to avoid the dreaded abandonment, but in the end, it erodes the trust and freedom necessary for love to grow.

3. Self-Annulment and Personal Sacrifice

One of the most evident characteristics of an emotionally dependent relationship is the tendency toward personal sacrifice and self-annulment. The dependent person is willing to set aside their own needs, desires, and values just to maintain the relationship. The idea of losing the partner is so frightening that any compromise seems acceptable, even if it involves a deep renunciation of one's identity.

In this context, love becomes an act of submission. The emotionally dependent person convinces themselves that to be loved, they must always be available, always ready to fulfill the partner's desires, even at the cost of their own well-being. Every conflict or divergence is avoided because asserting their needs might destabilize the relationship. This leads to a form of self-silencing, where the individual no longer expresses their authentic emotions but lives in function of the other.

However, this personal sacrifice never leads to happiness or security. On the contrary, the more the person annuls themselves, the more frustration and emptiness grow. The relationship becomes a golden cage, where love exists only on the condition that a part of the self is relinquished. The balance breaks, and love turns into a form of dependency where the partner becomes the only source of security and worth.

4. The Need for Constant Reassurance

Another distinctive feature of an emotionally dependent relationship is the constant need for reassurance. The dependent person never truly feels safe in the emotional bond, even when the partner shows love and affection. Every day, every moment, feels like there is a new test to pass, a new confirmation to obtain to feel loved and accepted.

This relentless search for reassurance can manifest through continuous questions: "Do you still love me?" "Why didn't you call me right away?" "Do you miss me when we're apart?" These questions are not simple curiosities but reflect deep insecurity, a constant fear that the partner might suddenly change their mind or stop loving them. Even when the partner offers sincere reassurances, they are never enough. The need resurfaces soon after, like a thirst that cannot be quenched.

Over time, the partner may feel suffocated by these continuous requests. The relationship becomes an emotional battlefield where every gesture or word must be carefully calibrated to avoid triggering the dependent person's anxiety. This creates tension and distance, further exacerbating the dependent person's insecurity, and the cycle repeats itself.

5. Difficulty Managing Conflict

Emotionally dependent relationships are often characterized by a deep difficulty in managing conflict. The dependent person sees conflict as a threat to the stability of the relationship. Every disagreement, every argument is perceived as a sign that something is going wrong, triggering anxiety about being abandoned. For this reason, conflicts are avoided or minimized at all costs, even when they are necessary for the relationship to grow and mature.

However, avoiding conflict does not mean resolving it. In fact, not addressing problems creates an accumulation of frustration, misunderstandings, and tensions that, over time, can explode in destructive ways. The inability to handle conflict in a healthy and constructive way is another sign of emotional dependency because the dependent person tends to sacrifice their voice and needs to avoid the risk of a confrontation that could end the relationship.

This dynamic often leads to a sense of resentment on the part of the partner, who may feel ignored or suffocated by the other's inability to discuss openly. In turn, the emotionally dependent person may feel misunderstood, constantly torn between the need to keep the peace and the growing frustration of not seeing their own needs recognized.

6. Idealization of the Partner

In emotionally dependent relationships, there is often a strong idealization of the partner. The dependent person tends to see the other not for who they truly are, with their flaws and vulnerabilities, but as a sort of savior, an emotional anchor who can offer security, unconditional love, and protection. This idealization reflects the desperate need to feel loved and accepted and often leads to a distorted view of reality.

Idealization can push the dependent person to ignore warning signs in the relationship, such as toxic behaviors or the partner's disinterest. Every flaw is minimized or justified because the idea of losing the partner is too painful to face. In this way, the dependent person finds themselves trapped in a relationship where the other is placed on a pedestal, and any flaw or failure is perceived as an existential threat.

Conclusion

Emotionally dependent relationships are steeped in fear, need, and sacrifice. The dependent person constantly lives with the anxiety of being abandoned, trying to control the partner and sacrificing themselves to maintain the relationship. The need for reassurance becomes relentless, and conflict is avoided at all costs out of fear of destabilizing the fragile emotional balance. At the root of all this lies deep insecurity, a wound that drives the individual to seek in the other a salvation that, however, can never truly be found.

The way out of these complex and painful dynamics lies in awareness and personal growth. Only by learning to recognize their own needs, cultivate self-esteem, and develop the ability to love without depending on the other can one build healthy relationships based on mutual love and freedom, where the person is seen and loved for who they are, not for what they can offer as a source of reassurance and stability.

The Roles of Victim and Perpetrator in Toxic Relationships Toxic relationships resemble an intense drama played out behind the scenes of an apparent love, where the roles of victim and perpetrator intertwine and often shift fluidly, in ways that are invisible to the outside. In these relationships, dynamics of power and control, paired with emotional suffering and manipulation, create a destructive cycle. The lines between who inflicts pain and who endures it often blur, as these roles are not always fixed. The victim, seemingly at the mercy of the perpetrator, may also participate in a dance of co-dependence, unintentionally reinforcing the dynamics of abuse and suffering.

The Victim: The Trap of Pain and Self-Sacrifice

In toxic relationships, the victim constantly lives in pain and anguish, desperately trying to save the relationship or rescue themselves from emotional or physical abuse. The victim is often someone who has developed deep insecurity and a sense of inadequacy. Behind a facade of strength or endurance lies an unhealed emotional wound—the belief of not being enough, of not deserving better love, and thus, being trapped in a relationship where pain is justified, or worse, deserved.

The victim clings to the relationship with the hope that things will change, that the partner (the perpetrator) will finally recognize their worth and begin to treat them with the respect and love they desperately seek. This often leads to extreme self-sacrifice, where the person completely erases themselves to please the other, believing that if they do enough, if they are perfect, the partner will stop inflicting pain. This self-sacrifice is one of the defining traits of the victim in toxic relationships:

they are willing to tolerate abuse, criticism, and manipulation to maintain the emotional connection, even if it is destructive.

At the heart of the victim lies a tragic hope—a blind faith that love can redeem even the worst of abusers. But this hope is what fuels the toxic cycle, as the victim becomes trapped in a spiral where every act of violence or manipulation is justified as a temporary mistake or a crisis that will eventually be resolved. The victim tends to idealize the partner, focusing on the rare moments of affection or attention they receive, downplaying the pain and justifying the abuse with excuses that become part of a self-saving narrative: "He does it because he loves me too much" or "He's not always like this, sometimes he's sweet."

This denial mechanism is what keeps the victim tied to the perpetrator. Each time the relationship seems irreparably broken, a small gesture of love, a promise of change, or a brief reconciliation reignites the hope that things can improve. However, this cycle of abuse and reconciliation is merely an illusion, and the victim ends up losing themselves in a maze of suffering and self-deception.

The Perpetrator: The Dominion of Abuse and Control

The perpetrator's role in toxic relationships is often seen as the one who wields power through control, manipulation, and sometimes violence. However, the perpetrator is not always the obvious monster one might expect. Often, they wear a mask of affection, love, or protection, disguising their need to dominate and control the other with gestures that may seem caring or protective. In fact, the perpetrator feeds off the power they hold over the victim, thriving on their ability to manipulate emotions, to make them feel loved one moment and utterly dependent the next.

Emotional control is one of the perpetrator's main tools. Through subtle manipulations, such as guilt-tripping, isolation, or gaslighting (a form of psychological abuse where the victim's perception of reality is distorted), the perpetrator keeps the victim trapped in a cycle of insecurity and dependence. Whenever the victim tries to rebel or assert their independence, the perpetrator responds with emotional attacks designed to destroy their self-esteem, making them feel small, weak, and incapable of living without them.

Gaslighting, in particular, is one of the most devastating tactics used by the perpetrator. Through distorting reality, the perpetrator convinces the victim that their feelings and perceptions are invalid. Phrases like "That never happened," "You're exaggerating," or "You imagined it" gradually lead the victim to doubt themselves, no longer trusting their own judgment, and relying solely on the partner to interpret reality. This creates a deep psychological dependence, where the victim feels lost without the perpetrator and becomes unable to distinguish right from wrong, just from unjust.

However, the perpetrator is not always fully aware of their role. Often, those who act as perpetrators in toxic relationships are themselves victims of unresolved trauma or dysfunctional relational patterns learned in childhood. Emotional co-dependence, fueled by unresolved insecurities and fears, drives the perpetrator to maintain control over the other as a way of avoiding their own pain and vulnerability. Paradoxically, the perpetrator is also trapped in the toxic relationship, unable to confront their need for power and control.

The Cycle of Violence: An Endless Tango

Toxic relationships often follow a repeating cycle of violence, trapping both partners in a dance of pain and reconciliation. This cycle begins with a phase of growing tension, where the perpetrator starts showing signs of frustration, irritability, and control. The victim, in an attempt to avoid conflict or placate the partner, begins to act submissively, trying to prevent the eruption of violence.

This phase is followed by an explosion of violence, which can be emotional, verbal, physical, or psychological. The perpetrator unleashes their anger, frustration, or need for dominance on the victim, inflicting pain and humiliation. The victim, paralyzed by fear and confusion, passively endures or tries to fight back but is never able to truly break the cycle.

After the violent phase, comes the reconciliation phase. The perpetrator may appear remorseful, apologizing or promising that "it will never happen again." In this phase, the victim, desperate to believe that their partner can change, accepts the apologies, hoping that this time the change will be real. This phase is highly manipulative, as the promise of change or redemption merely keeps the victim's hope alive, feeding the toxic cycle.

Finally, the cycle concludes with a phase of apparent calm, where the relationship seems to recover. The partners may experience moments of peace, of affection, but beneath the surface, the ground is fragile, and the tension begins to build again, setting the stage for the next explosion of violence.

Role Reversal: The Victim Becomes the Perpetrator

In many toxic relationships, the roles of victim and perpetrator are not fixed. Often, role reversals occur, where the victim may turn into the perpetrator, and the perpetrator may, in turn, feel like the victim. This happens because both partners are trapped in a dynamic of pain, fear, and need that drives them to react dysfunctionally.

The victim, after enduring repeated abuse, may start exhibiting toxic behaviors themselves, such as emotional manipulation or emotional blackmail, in an attempt to defend themselves or regain a sense of power. Similarly, the perpetrator, when the victim withdraws or rebels, may feel abandoned or rejected, taking on the role of the victim and trying to justify their abusive behaviors as a reaction to their own suffering.

This dance of roles makes toxic relationships extremely complex and difficult to break, as both parties end up reinforcing the dynamic of abuse without clearly seeing who is inflicting or enduring the pain.

Conclusion

The roles of victim and perpetrator in toxic relationships are two sides of the same coin, bound by a thin thread of fear, insecurity, and manipulation. Both roles fuel a destructive cycle that repeats itself, trapping both partners in a relationship that gradually erodes their self-esteem and freedom. Breaking this cycle requires deep self-awareness and recognition of one's worth, as well as the courage to acknowledge the toxicity of the relationship and take the necessary steps to escape.

Healthy relationships are built on reciprocity, respect, and freedom, not power and control. Leaving a toxic relationship means finding oneself again, rebuilding one's identity, and learning to live love not as dependence but as a conscious and authentic choice.

Cycles of Dependency: Attraction, Idealization, Disillusionment, and Dependency Emotionally dependent relationships follow a repetitive, pervasive cycle that engulfs partners in an emotional vortex filled with intense feelings, unrealistic expectations, and a growing inability to detach from a bond that, rather than nourishing, ends up consuming. This cycle of dependency is not linear but cyclical and relentless, moving through four main phases: attraction, idealization, disillusionment, and, ultimately, dependency. Each of these phases has its own power, its own dynamics, and inevitably leads to the creation of a bond where love is confused with necessity, and need is mistaken for feeling.

1. Attraction: The Illusion of Love at First Sight

It all begins with attraction. In this phase, two people meet and feel an immediate connection. This connection can be chemical, emotional, or even spiritual. It is the moment when the heart races, thoughts become lighter, and everything seems to fall into place. However, attraction is not just physical; it is also the feeling of being found, of finally meeting someone who "completes" what was missing. There is intense excitement surrounding each encounter, and the mind begins projecting images of what this new relationship could be. The other person is perceived as special, unique, and a sense of exclusivity quickly develops, reinforcing the emerging bond.

But attraction, in an emotionally dependent relationship, is more than just a game of feelings. It is the beginning of a search for completeness, where the other is not just someone to fall in love with but the solution to an inner void that the emotionally dependent person seeks to fill. In this phase, the emotionally dependent person is overwhelmed by the hope that this time, this relationship, will be the answer to all their unresolved emotional needs. The new partner is seen as the missing emotional anchor, and this perception amplifies the intensity of the attraction.

However, this strong initial attraction is not without danger. This is where the idealization process begins, where the other is invested with an almost salvific role, and the emotionally dependent person clings to the illusion that this connection can finally heal every emotional wound, solve every insecurity.

2. Idealization: The Other as Savior

In the second phase of the dependency cycle, attraction turns into idealization. The partner is placed on a pedestal and seen as the perfect person, the ideal companion embodying all the desired qualities. Every gesture, every word from the other is interpreted as confirmation of the depth of the bond, and flaws, if they exist, are minimized or completely ignored. At this point, the relationship seems pure and perfect, without shadows or conflicts.

Idealization, however, is a form of illusion. The emotionally dependent person projects all their desires and unrealistic expectations onto the partner. The other becomes a sort of emotional savior, the answer to a deep need for love and acceptance that has never been met. This phase is fueled by the belief that love—true love—must be overwhelming, all-encompassing, and perfect. The partner becomes the sole beacon in a sea of emotional uncertainties, and the emotionally dependent person pours all their energy into keeping this idealized image alive.

This idealization leads to emotional fusion, where the emotionally dependent person gradually loses touch with themselves. There are no longer boundaries between themselves and the other: the partner's needs, desires, and feelings become primary, while their own are relegated to the background. Love, at this stage, is experienced as a symbiosis, a union that gives a sense of completeness but is, in reality, fragile and destined to collapse under the weight of unrealistic expectations.

3. Disillusionment: Reality Unfolds

The third phase of the cycle is disillusionment. After the intensity of attraction and the bliss of idealization, comes the moment when reality begins to break through. The partner's flaws, previously ignored or minimized, become evident. Small signs of incompatibility, differences in desires and needs, start to surface. What was once idealized is now seen with more critical eyes, and the emotionally dependent person begins to feel betrayed.

This phase is particularly painful because the partner, who was once seen as perfect, now seems to fall short of expectations. The other, who was supposed to be the answer to all insecurities, turns out to be unable to fill that inner void. Disillusionment is accompanied by a sense of loss, confusion, and often anger. The emotionally dependent person wonders what went wrong, why the initial magic has dissipated, and may start blaming themselves or the partner for this failure.

Disillusionment is not only the recognition of the other's flaws but also the awakening of old emotional wounds. The insecurities and fears that were temporarily set aside during the idealization phase return with full force. The emotionally dependent person may feel abandoned again, rejected, or not enough, and this reawakens anxiety and the need for reassurance. However, instead of addressing these emotions in a healthy way, the emotionally dependent person clings even more desperately to the relationship, hoping it can return to the initial perfection.

4. Dependency: The Trap of Obsessive Need

The final phase of the cycle is true dependency. After attraction, idealization, and disillusionment, the emotionally dependent person finds themselves trapped in a bond they cannot break, despite the pain and frustration. At this stage, the relationship is no longer experienced as a conscious choice but as a necessity. The other becomes a kind of emotional drug, a presence that cannot be lived without, even if it no longer brings joy or fulfillment.

In dependency, the partner is perceived as essential to one's emotional existence. The thought of losing the other triggers deep anguish, a sense of emptiness that feels unbearable. The emotionally dependent person clings to the bond with all their strength, desperately trying to recapture the intensity and security of the relationship's early stages. However, this search is doomed to fail because the relationship, at this point, is already compromised by toxic dynamics and unrealistic expectations.

Emotional dependency leads to a spiral of control, jealousy, and constant need for reassurance. The emotionally dependent person may try to manipulate the partner, holding onto them with extreme gestures or emotional blackmail to avoid being abandoned. Every moment of distance, every action that does not meet expectations, is seen as a threat, and the relationship becomes an emotional prison, where both partners are trapped.

But dependency never leads to true satisfaction. The emotionally dependent person lives in a state of frustration and suffering because what they are seeking—unconditional love and emotional security—cannot be found externally but only through an internal process of awareness and healing. The relationship, therefore, becomes a source of anxiety and torment rather than joy and mutual growth.

Conclusion: The Endless Cycle

The cycle of attraction, idealization, disillusionment, and dependency repeats itself endlessly in emotionally dependent relationships, creating a bond that, instead of liberating, imprisons. Each time the cycle completes, it begins again, with new hopes, new illusions, and a growing inability to break free from the bond. The emotionally dependent person finds themselves searching in the other for what they should find within themselves: self-esteem, security, and personal worth.

The way out of this cycle requires deep self-awareness and a journey of personal growth. Only by recognizing one's need for dependency and learning to cultivate self-love can one break the cycle and build healthier relationships based on reciprocity, freedom, and mutual respect. For love to be true, it cannot be an emotional prison but must be a space where both partners feel free to be themselves—without fear, without control, and without the need to fill voids that only authenticity and awareness can fill.

Co-Dependence: When Both Partners Are Emotionally Dependent

Co-dependence is an emotional dance in which two partners, both trapped in their insecurities and unresolved needs, entwine themselves in a seemingly unbreakable web of emotions. It is a relationship where love becomes confused with dependence, where each partner seeks validation from the other, while simultaneously sustaining a toxic dynamic of control and sacrifice. In a co-dependent relationship, both partners are emotionally dependent on each other, and this interdependence not only binds them together but also imprisons them in a cycle of mutual need, fear, and self-denial.

Emotional Symbiosis: When the Other Becomes Everything

In co-dependence, both partners are caught in a kind of emotional symbiosis where one cannot exist without the other. Their identities are no longer separate but entwined in a way that seems inseparable. Instead of being complete individuals who meet to share part of their lives, co-dependent partners become each other's lifeblood, a source of security, comfort, and sometimes emotional salvation. However, this relationship is not based on reciprocity or unconditional love, but on mutual psychological dependence.

Each partner clings to the other like an anchor, unable to imagine life without them. It's as if the other person is the only source of stability, and without that constant presence, everything would collapse into an unbearable void. Love, in this context, is no longer a choice but a necessity: it's as though both partners need to stay together despite the pain, because separation would mean confronting their fears and insecurities without the other's support. In this way, co-dependence is not just an emotional bond but a kind of emotional prison where the partner is not just someone to love but a vital survival anchor.

The Need to Save and Be Saved

One of the hallmarks of co-dependence is the mutual need to save and be saved. Often, one partner takes on the role of the "savior," someone who tries to fix the other's problems, heal their emotional wounds, and protect them from pain. This partner, whom we can call the "savior," feels responsible for the other's happiness and well-being, and this responsibility becomes a mission that gives meaning to their existence. They continually sacrifice their own needs, dreams, and desires to try to repair what is broken in their partner.

On the other hand, there is the "needy" partner, who takes on the role of the one who must be cared for, nurtured, and protected. This partner leans entirely on the other, depending on them not only for emotional support but also for their own identity. They convince themselves that without the other, they would not survive, that the other is the only one who can understand their suffering and provide the unconditional love they need.

However, this dynamic is far from balanced. The savior, in trying to heal the other, ends up suffocating them, while the needy partner becomes increasingly dependent and unable to face their own challenges independently. This creates a vicious cycle where both partners are locked in a dance where the savior keeps giving, and the needy partner keeps taking, without either being able to grow or change.

Paradoxically, even the "savior" is dependent. Their identity is tied to the need to be necessary, to be the hero who saves the other. If the needy partner were to heal, the savior would lose their purpose. In this way, both partners keep the dependency dynamics alive, as each needs the other to justify their own existence.

Control and Jealousy as Manifestations of Fear

In co-dependence, control plays a crucial role. Both partners, consciously or unconsciously, try to control the other to prevent the relationship from changing or ending. This control manifests in various ways, from jealousy to obsessiveness to emotional manipulation. The savior tries to control the needy partner to ensure that they don't "slip away," that they continue to depend on them. The needy partner, on the other hand, may try to maintain emotional control over the savior through vulnerability and a constant need for reassurance.

Jealousy often reflects the fear of losing the other. Since both partners see themselves as incapable of living without the other, any sign of distance or interest in other people is perceived as an existential threat. The savior may become jealous of the needy partner's friendships, fearing that someone else might provide the support they need. Similarly, the needy partner may fear that the savior, tired of carrying the weight of the relationship, might seek comfort or relief elsewhere.

This dynamic of control and jealousy not only erodes mutual trust but also prevents each partner from developing healthy emotional independence. Both are so focused on keeping the relationship intact that they fail to see how stifling and damaging it has become to their personal growth.

The Denial of Personal Needs

In a co-dependent relationship, both partners deny their own personal needs in favor of the other's or, more precisely, in favor of what they perceive as the necessity of keeping the relationship alive at all costs. The savior gives up their desires, dreams, and needs to focus on the partner, believing that this sacrifice is necessary to hold the relationship together. The needy partner, in turn, may suppress their genuine needs for fear of losing the savior's approval, living in accordance with the other's expectations.

This self-denial not only creates deep emotional frustration but further feeds mutual dependence. Since neither partner feels free to express their desires or needs, the relationship becomes a closed loop where dysfunctional dynamics reinforce one another. There is no room for individual growth or freedom because both partners are trapped in a relationship where one's emotional survival depends on the presence of the other.

In this denial of personal needs, both partners end up living a "half-life." Rather than face the pain of separation, they accept living in continual sacrifice without ever reaching true emotional fulfillment. This can lead to an accumulation of resentment, even if hidden, as both partners feel, deep down, that they are not living authentically but are prisoners of dependency dynamics.

The Endless Cycle of Pain and Reconciliation

As with toxic relationships, co-dependence also develops a continuous cycle of conflict and reconciliation. Since the relationship is not based on true reciprocity but on dysfunctional dynamics, conflicts are inevitable. Both partners find themselves living through moments of crisis where frustration and pain rise to the surface. However, the fear of losing the other and facing emotional solitude pushes both to seek reconciliation.

This reconciliation, however, never truly resolves the underlying problems. Instead, it becomes a sort of temporary truce where both partners deceive themselves into thinking things can improve. But since the relationship continues to be based on emotional dependency, the cycle of conflict and reconciliation repeats endlessly, trapping both in a spiral of pain that seems to have no end.

The Path to Healing: Recognizing Co-Dependence

Breaking free from a co-dependent relationship is difficult, but not impossible. The first step toward healing is recognizing the nature of co-dependence, understanding how the dynamics of need and control are destroying the possibility of authentic love. Both partners must confront their deepest fears: the fear of being alone, the fear of not being enough, the fear of not being loved.

The healing process requires deep inner reflection and often external support, such as therapy. Both partners must learn to emotionally detach from one another, develop their own autonomous identities, and cultivate self-love without constantly seeking validation from the other.

Only when each partner can love and respect themselves for who they are—without feeling trapped in dynamics of need and control—can the relationship transform into a healthy bond based on freedom, reciprocity, and mutual respect. Co-dependence can be broken, but it requires courage, awareness, and the genuine desire to live a truer, freer love.

Conclusion

Co-dependence is an emotional trap in which both partners, despite loving each other, bind themselves in a dynamic of mutual need that stifles individual growth and authenticity. Each seeks in the other what they should find within themselves: security, worth, and love. But instead of nourishing each other, they consume themselves in a cycle of control, sacrifice, and frustration.

Recognizing co-dependence and having the courage to face it is the first step toward healing. Only when both partners are able to live and love autonomously can the relationship transform into a healthy bond where love is not a dependency but a free and reciprocal choice.

Part 2: Recognizing Emotional DependencyChapter 4Warning Signs of Emotional Dependency

Emotional dependency is a subtle trap, a condition that slowly creeps into a person's life, often masked by the intensity of love and devotion to the other. At first, the bond may seem simply deep and passionate, but over time, warning signs begin to emerge, revealing that what seemed like a relationship based on love has turned into an emotional prison. Emotional dependency manifests through behaviors and dynamics that, once recognized, clearly indicate that love is no longer a choice but an obsessive need.

1 **Constant Fear of Abandonment** One of the most evident signs of emotional dependency is the constant fear of abandonment. The dependent person lives with the perpetual anxiety that the other might leave them, even when there are no concrete signs of withdrawal. Every gesture, word, or action of the partner is scrutinized for clues that confirm or dispel this fear. An unanswered message, a colder-than-usual tone of voice, or a change in habits can trigger deep anxiety in the dependent person.

This fear of abandonment leads to a constant search for reassurance. The emotionally dependent person needs to frequently hear phrases like "I love you" or "I will never leave you," and even when these words are spoken, they are never enough. The fear soon returns, pushing the dependent person to seek further confirmation and live in a state of continuous uncertainty.

2 **Self-Effacement and Extreme Sacrifice** Another crucial sign of emotional dependency is the renunciation of one's own needs and desires. The dependent person begins to constantly put the other's needs above their own, ignoring their own desires, dreams, and even well-being. This sacrifice is not a conscious choice of generosity or unconditional love, but a necessity rooted in the fear that if they do not do enough for the partner, they risk being abandoned.

Extreme sacrifice can manifest in various ways: accepting unsatisfying living conditions, giving up personal goals to support the partner, or even tolerating harmful or abusive behaviors just to maintain the relationship. This self-effacement is a clear sign that the relationship is no longer based on reciprocity but has become a form of emotional submission where the dependent person lives to please the other, fearing that asserting their own needs might cause everything to fall apart.

3 **Obsessive Jealousy and Control** A frequent warning sign of emotional dependency is obsessive jealousy. The dependent person constantly fears that the partner might find someone else, even when there are no concrete

reasons to suspect it. This jealousy is not just an occasional concern but an obsession that can consume the individual. Every interaction the partner has with the outside world, every relationship, friendship, or social contact is perceived as a potential threat.

This jealousy often translates into controlling behavior. The dependent person tries to monitor every aspect of the partner's life, from checking messages and phone calls to keeping track of movements and meetings. This control does not stem from distrust of the partner but from deep internal insecurity. The dependent person feels that if they do not have total control over the relationship, the other might slip away, and so they become obsessively vigilant, constantly seeking confirmations and reassurances.

4 **Social Isolation** Another alarming sign of emotional dependency is social isolation. In an attempt to devote themselves entirely to the relationship, the dependent person may progressively distance themselves from friends, family, and all other important relationships. Often, this happens unconsciously: time and energy are entirely dedicated to the partner, and all other relationships are relegated to the background.

Isolation may also be fueled by the fear that other people might criticize the relationship or question the partner's behavior. The dependent person prefers to avoid situations where they might feel vulnerable or receive negative judgments about the relationship. In the end, the bond with the partner becomes the sole focal point of life, and this isolation only intensifies the dependency, as the person finds themselves without other emotional or social supports to rely on.

5 **Lack of Boundaries** In healthy relationships, there are clear boundaries between partners: each has their own personal space, their own interests, and the right to maintain a certain level of autonomy. In emotional dependency, these boundaries dissolve. The dependent person struggles to establish clear limits and often accepts behaviors that should not be tolerated just to avoid conflicts or abandonment.

The lack of boundaries manifests when the dependent person allows the partner to invade every aspect of their life, accepting conditions that undermine their dignity and well-being. They may agree to do things they do not want to do or tolerate controlling and manipulative behaviors just to avoid questioning the relationship. This sign is particularly insidious because the emotionally dependent person often does not realize how much they are sacrificing themselves until the emotional damage becomes too great.

6 **Obsessive Need for Reassurance** In emotional dependency, there is a constant and obsessive need for reassurance. The dependent person never feels truly secure in the relationship and needs to continuously hear that the partner loves them and will not leave them. This need manifests in constant requests for confirmation: "Do you still love me?", "What do you feel for me?", "You'll never leave me, right?".

Even when the partner responds positively to these requests, the relief is only temporary. Soon after, the dependent person feels anxious again, as if the other's love is precarious, ready to vanish. This incessant need for confirmation only fuels the dependency, as the emotionally dependent person lives in a state of constant uncertainty, desperately trying to maintain emotional control over the relationship.

7 **Inability to Leave the Relationship Despite the Pain** One of the strongest signs of emotional dependency is the inability to leave the relationship, even when it causes suffering. The dependent person is willing to endure painful, humiliating, or toxic situations just to avoid facing the fear of loneliness or abandonment. Despite being aware that the relationship is no longer healthy, that conflicts are constant, and that happiness seems increasingly distant, the emotionally dependent person cannot break away.

This behavior results from the fear of loss and the inability to imagine life without the partner. The relationship, even if painful, is perceived as the only source of emotional security, and the dependent person prefers to remain trapped in the pain rather than face the uncertainty of the future. This leads to a cycle of suffering where, despite the desire to be happy, the fear of being alone prevails.

8 **Dependence on the Partner's Presence and Attention** Finally, a clear sign of emotional dependency is total dependence on the partner's presence and attention. The dependent person does not feel complete or fulfilled unless they are constantly in the partner's company. Every moment spent away from the other is filled with anxiety, and any activity that does not involve the partner seems meaningless.

This extreme need for closeness can lead to emotional fusion, where the dependent person gradually loses touch with their own interests and identity. The relationship becomes the sole source of meaning in life, and without the constant presence of the other, the emotionally dependent person feels empty, worthless, and lost.

Conclusion

The warning signs of emotional dependency are numerous, and if left unrecognized, they can drag a person into a spiral of suffering and self-effacement. Emotional dependency is not simply intense love but a condition where the other becomes an emotional necessity, and the relationship is experienced as the only source of security and personal value.

Recognizing these signs is the first step toward awareness and healing. Only through a process of inner reflection and personal growth can one break the cycle of emotional dependency and build relationships based on autonomy, reciprocity, and authentic love, where both partners are free to be themselves without the need to control or be controlled.

Emotional and Behavioral Symptoms of Emotional Dependency: Jealousy, Control, Need for Reassurance

Emotional dependency is an emotional whirlwind that distorts how we live and perceive love, turning what should be a free expression of affection into a web of fears, insecurities, and compulsive behaviors. Among the most evident symptoms of this psychological and emotional state are jealousy, control, and the constant need for reassurance. These symptoms, which may sometimes seem like minor initial signs, intensify over time, engulfing the individual in a spiral of anxiety and obsession, poisoning the relationship itself.

Jealousy: The Shadow of the Fear of Losing the Other

Jealousy is one of the most frequent and corrosive symptoms of emotional dependency. In a healthy relationship, there may be natural concern or slight insecurity related to third parties, but in emotional dependency, jealousy turns into an obsession, a constant shadow that follows every gesture and thought.The emotionally dependent person lives in constant fear that their partner may cheat, leave, or be attracted to someone else. This fear is not rational, nor is it based on concrete events, but it stems from deep inner insecurity. It is a projection of their own fears of not being enough, of not being loved as desired, and of being replaced. Even a simple smile from the partner toward another person or an innocent conversation can trigger a disproportionate reaction of anxiety and jealousy.In these cases, jealousy becomes an obsessive presence, a fixed thought that disturbs both mind and heart. Every social occasion, every meeting with friends or colleagues, is experienced as a potential threat. The dependent partner may begin controlling every detail, asking persistently about who the partner saw, where they were, and who they spoke with. However, the real root of this jealousy is not external; it does not involve the partner's behavior but rather stems from internal emotional fragility. The emotionally dependent person, unable to fully trust themselves and their worth, projects all their insecurities onto the other, seeing every small crack in the relationship as a potential escape route for the partner.This jealousy is paralyzing, both for the person experiencing it and for the one enduring it. The jealous partner constantly lives on the edge of suspicion, and the other feels suffocated by the control, which only increases emotional distance.

Control: The Need to Dominate the Bond

At the heart of jealousy lies control, another crucial symptom of emotional dependency. Control is not a manifestation of strength but a reaction to the deep fear of losing the other. The emotionally dependent person feels the need to monitor every aspect of their partner's life to feel secure in the relationship. However, this security is merely an illusion, as control only further feeds their insecurity and fragility.Control can manifest in different ways. Some behaviors are subtle, like wanting to know who the partner is with or where they are or constantly asking to be informed about every detail of the day. Others are more evident and invasive, such as checking the partner's phone messages, demanding explanations for every interaction with others, or trying to limit the partner's social outings to avoid potential "temptations." These behaviors create an unhealthy power dynamic within the relationship, where the dependent partner tries to gain full control over the other, hoping this will guarantee the stability of the bond.In reality, control never leads to the sought-after security. In fact, the more one tries to control the other, the more the partner feels suffocated and tends to distance themselves. This distancing only fuels the emotionally dependent person's fear, who, in response, tries to intensify control, creating a vicious cycle of mistrust and fear.In a healthy relationship, clear boundaries exist between partners, and each is free to maintain their own identity and autonomy. In emotional dependency, however, these boundaries are eroded, as the dependent person perceives separation as a threat, unable to see that true love grows in freedom, not in constraint.

Obsessive Need for Reassurance: A Void That Is Never Filled

The need for reassurance is another hallmark symptom of emotional dependency. The dependent person never feels fully secure in their partner's love and affection, even when it is clearly demonstrated. It is as if every reassurance fades almost immediately, leaving room for a new wave of insecurity. Words of love and affectionate gestures, which in a healthy relationship would be enough to make someone feel loved and appreciated, are never enough. There is an inner void that seems impossible to fill, an anxiety that keeps returning, demanding more.The emotionally dependent person may continuously ask their partner to repeat their love, with phrases like: "Do you still love me?", "Do you really desire me?", "Do you miss me when we're not together?", or "You won't leave me, right?" Even if the partner responds sincerely, this brings no lasting relief, as the root of that obsessive need is not found in the other's actions but in a lack of self-esteem and internal security. This constant search for reassurance not only emotionally exhausts the person asking but also the one receiving these questions. The emotionally dependent partner may feel continually tested, as if they must prove their love anew every day, and this can generate frustration and emotional distance. The paradox is that the more the emotionally dependent person seeks reassurance, the more they push the other away, as the relationship becomes an emotional burden rather than a source of joy and connection. The need for reassurance expresses an internal lack: the dependent person seeks from the other a security they cannot find within themselves. It is like trying to fill a leaky bucket: no matter how much water is poured in, it will never fill until the hole at the bottom is fixed. In the case of emotional dependency, this hole is the lack of self-esteem and self-love. The emotionally dependent person never feels enough and constantly seeks from their partner confirmation that they are loved, desired, and important. But the love of others can never compensate for the lack of love for oneself.

The Common Root: The Fear of Not Being Loved

Behind jealousy, control, and the need for reassurance lies a deep and universal fear: the fear of not being loved, the belief that if they do not do enough, the other may leave, leaving behind an unbearable void. The emotionally dependent person does not believe they are worthy of love for who they are but thinks they must constantly "earn" love through sacrifice, dedication, or control. This fear leads to a destructive relational dynamic, where love becomes a struggle for emotional survival. Every gesture of the other is interpreted through the filter of insecurity, and every distance is experienced as a sign of imminent rejection or abandonment. To escape this cycle of suffering, deep self-work is necessary. Healing from emotional dependency begins with awareness of these symptoms and the understanding that true love can never be born from fear, control, or incessant requests for reassurance. It is a long journey, made up of introspection, self-care, and often therapeutic support, but it is the only way to transform a relationship of dependency into one based on respect, freedom, and authentic love.

Conclusion

The emotional and behavioral symptoms of emotional dependency—jealousy, control, and the need for reassurance—are signs that something in the way we experience love is profoundly distorted. These symptoms arise from fear, insecurity, and a lack of trust in oneself. The emotionally dependent person seeks in the other a stability they cannot find within themselves, but this search only drives them further away from true love, which can only exist in freedom and mutual trust.

Obsession with the Partner: Intrusive Thoughts and Fear of Loneliness

Love, when healthy, is a flame that illuminates without burning, warming without consuming. However, when it turns into obsession, love loses its gentle light and becomes a fire that devours, consuming every thought and emotion until life becomes a prison of anxiety, desire, and fear. Obsession with the partner is a journey toward self-dissolution, where the heart, instead of being free to love, is trapped in an invisible web of intrusive thoughts and the paralyzing fear of loneliness.

The Siege of Intrusive Thoughts

Obsession with the partner is like a fog that invades every corner of the mind, suffocating the ability to think clearly and live peacefully. Intrusive thoughts become a constant presence, a sort of mental background accompanying every moment of the day. These thoughts are unwanted, but they creep in without warning, disrupting even the simplest activities. While working, reading, or talking to friends, the mind continually returns to the object of the obsession: the partner.Intrusive thoughts are obsessive, repetitive, and often distressing. They can concern where the partner is, who they are with, what they are doing, or even doubts about the sincerity of their feelings. Every little detail, even the most trivial, becomes the subject of speculation and analysis: "Why

didn't they respond right away?" "What does that silence mean?" "Why did they look at that person like that?" The emotionally dependent person's mind is a prison where every thought transforms into self-feeding anxiety.These obsessive thoughts offer no respite, and the person finds themselves living in a state of emotional hyper-vigilance, where every slight variation in the partner's behavior is interpreted as a possible sign of distancing or abandonment. Even a simple delay in responding to a message can become a source of worry, triggering a chain of intrusive thoughts: "Maybe they don't love me anymore," "Maybe they've met someone else," "What did I do wrong?" Every small crack in communication becomes a giant rift, capable of sinking the entire relationship.This obsession also extends to when the partner is not physically present. The absence, even temporary, is experienced with disproportionate emotional intensity, as if the relationship itself is constantly in jeopardy. The obsessed person cannot mentally detach from the partner, living in a perpetual state of emotional alertness. Every moment apart becomes a mental torment, a void that seems impossible to fill except through the constant presence of the loved one.

Fear of Loneliness: The Void That Frightens

At the root of obsession with the partner lies an even deeper and more visceral fear: the fear of loneliness. This fear is so intense and deeply rooted that it conditions every thought and action of the dependent person. Loneliness is not experienced as a temporary or natural state but as an unbearable condition, a void that drains all energy and leaves only a sense of anguish and despair.For those suffering from emotional dependency, loneliness is not merely the physical absence of the other but an existential lack. Without the partner, the person feels incomplete, devoid of purpose, as if their identity dissolves in the absence. The relationship thus becomes a refuge, an anchor of salvation, and the idea of losing it triggers a paralyzing fear. It's like standing on the edge of a cliff, with the sensation that if the other steps away even for a moment, one will fall into the abyss.The fear of loneliness pushes the obsessed person to do anything to keep the partner close, even at the cost of sacrificing their own dignity or well-being. They become willing to tolerate behaviors that, in a healthy emotional state, would be unacceptable, just to avoid facing the prospect of being alone. This fear fuels the obsession, as the dependent person lives with the constant anxiety that the partner might leave, and this thought is so unbearable that it leads to controlling or extremely dependent behaviors.Loneliness is not just experienced as a moment of physical isolation but as an emotional void. The dependent person has built their identity around the relationship, and the idea of being without the partner represents not only the loss of the other but also the loss of self. Without the partner, the dependent person no longer knows who they are, what they want, or how to manage their emotions. It's as if the relationship were the only fixed point in a sea of uncertainties and insecurities, and without it, they feel adrift, unable to face life alone.

Emotional Fusion and Loss of Self

Obsession with the partner leads to a form of emotional fusion, where the dependent person progressively loses touch with themselves. There are no longer personal desires, needs, or dreams: everything revolves around the other. They live for the other, through the other, and the idea of an independent life becomes inconceivable. In this state, the relationship is no longer a meeting between two distinct individuals but a sort of emotional symbiosis, where one completely depends on the other for emotional stability.This fusion results in a loss of autonomy and personal identity. The dependent person no longer sees themselves as an individual in their own right but only as part of a whole. Every decision, every thought, every action is subordinated to the presence and will of the partner. They become incapable of living individual experiences without feeling guilty or empty, as if every moment spent apart from the other were a threat to the very existence of the relationship.This loss of self is extremely damaging, as it deprives the person of the opportunity to grow, discover their potential, and live a full and satisfying life. The partner, in this context, is no longer seen as a life companion but as an emotional savior, a figure to cling to in order to avoid confronting one's own inner void.

Obsessive Behaviors and Cycles of Anxiety

Obsession with the partner also manifests through a series of obsessive behaviors, which can range from compulsive messaging to constantly seeking reassurance, to controlling the other's activities. These behaviors do not stem from a desire for love or affection but from the need to reduce the anxiety that arises from the fear of losing the partner or being abandoned.Every interaction becomes a test to pass, a check to see if the other is still involved and present. Every silence or delay is experienced with anguish, and every affectionate response provides temporary relief. However, this relief lasts only briefly, as the anxiety soon returns, pushing the obsessed person to seek further confirmations and reassurances.This creates a cycle of anxiety and relief that repeats endlessly. The mind cannot free itself from the idea that the partner might leave, and every gesture or word from the other is examined and interpreted through the lens of insecurity. This cycle is exhausting, both for the person experiencing it and for the partner, who constantly feels pressured to provide continuous confirmations to keep the other calm.

The Path to Healing: Recognizing the Obsession

The first step in overcoming obsession with the partner is recognizing it. Often, those who suffer from it are unaware that their love has turned into a form of obsessive dependency. They justify their behaviors with the intensity of their feelings or the fear of losing the other, but healthy love can never be an emotional prison.Healing requires deep inner work, leading to the rediscovery of oneself outside of the relationship. It is necessary to confront the fear of loneliness and learn to see one's own company as a value rather than a threat. Only through rebuilding self-esteem and discovering an autonomous and fulfilling life can one free themselves from obsession with the partner.Therapy can be a valuable tool in this process, as it allows for the exploration of the deep roots of emotional dependency and the development of new strategies to deal with anxiety and the fear of loneliness. Only by learning to live in harmony with oneself can one transform an obsessive relationship into a free and authentic love, where the partner is no longer a lifeline but a life companion with whom to grow and share, without fear and without dependency.

Conclusion

Obsession with the partner is a form of emotional imprisonment that feeds on intrusive thoughts and the fear of loneliness. In this state, love turns into dependency, and the relationship becomes a refuge to avoid confronting one's deepest insecurities and fears. The mind fills with doubts, anxiety grows, and the obsessed person loses touch with themselves, living only through their connection with the other.Overcoming obsession requires courage and introspection. It is a healing journey that involves rediscovering oneself and accepting loneliness as a natural part of life. Only when one learns to be comfortable with themselves can they experience authentic love, free from obsession and fear, where the partner is not an object of control but a companion on the journey of life.

Personal Sacrifice: Losing Oneself for the Other

There is a kind of love that is narrated through the language of sacrifice, a love that feeds on self-denial, extreme compromises, and constant self-renunciation. It is the love of those driven by a deep fear of losing the other or not being enough, who end up completely nullifying themselves for their partner. In this process, personal sacrifice becomes a daily act, a slow erosion of identity that, over time, leaves the person hollowed out, like a shadow of what they once were.Sacrificing for the other, when healthy, is a natural part of a couple's life. It involves the ability to adapt, to embrace the other's needs, and to compromise. But when this sacrifice turns into self-annihilation, it is no longer a choice but a necessity rooted in fear. It becomes an unconditional surrender of one's will, a continuous renunciation of one's essence and desires. This kind of sacrifice is not an expression of authentic love but rather an act of desperation, where one lives under the illusion that the only way to keep the partner close is to give up everything, even to the point of forgetting oneself entirely.

The Progressive Loss of Identity

In the early stages of a relationship based on emotional dependency, personal sacrifice can seem harmless, even natural. It starts with small gestures, like giving up a night out with friends to be with the partner or setting aside personal hobbies to accommodate the other's desires. These gestures, though seemingly trivial, mark the beginning of a progressive renunciation of one's identity.Over time, these small concessions become habits. Dreams and goals are put on the back burner, personal needs go unexpressed, and it is accepted that the partner's priorities always come before one's own. This process is often gradual and almost imperceptible, but it has a devastating impact. The person who sacrifices themselves for the other finds themselves living a life that no longer belongs to them, a life shaped exclusively by the desires and expectations of the partner.In this state, the dependent person's individuality slowly dissolves. There is no longer room for themselves, their interests, or their dreams. Every choice is made in function of the other, and every personal desire is shelved to avoid conflict or, worse yet, the risk of being abandoned. The person who sacrifices themselves lives with the belief that, to be loved, they must fully conform to the partner's needs, losing the ability to assert their own individuality.

Silencing Needs and Fear of Conflict

One of the most devastating consequences of personal sacrifice is the silencing of one's own needs. The person who nullifies themselves for the other no longer feels entitled to express their desires or needs. Every time an inner conflict arises, it is suppressed for fear that it might disturb the balance of the relationship. Every time they want to ask for something, they remain silent, hoping the other can intuit or understand without needing words.However, this silence is not a conscious choice but a consequence of the fear of conflict. The dependent person develops a distorted belief: they think that expressing their needs could lead to the end of the relationship, that any request or disagreement might drive the partner away. So, instead of affirming their feelings or desires, the person prefers to stifle their inner voice, constantly adapting to the other's will.This dynamic creates growing emotional tension. Even though needs are repressed, they do not disappear but accumulate beneath the surface. The person who sacrifices themselves for the other becomes increasingly frustrated and dissatisfied, but they cannot voice these emotions. This leads to hidden resentment, a silent suffering that grows over time but is never openly expressed.

Sacrifice as a Form of Control

Paradoxically, self-annihilation and personal sacrifice can become a form of control in the relationship. Although it may seem contradictory, those who sacrifice themselves for the other often unconsciously hope to gain something in return: love, gratitude, emotional security. The dependent person believes that if they do enough, if they are devoted enough, the partner will never leave. Sacrifice thus becomes a strategy to keep the partner attached, to ensure some form of recognition or emotional reward.However, this expectation is bound to lead to frustration and pain. True love cannot be bought through sacrifice, and the partner, instead of recognizing the sacrifice, may feel suffocated or even guilty. In this way, the relationship turns into an emotional trap, where personal sacrifice never leads to the desired security but only to a growing sense of frustration and bitterness.The control exercised through sacrifice is subtle but present. Every time a person gives up part of themselves, they hope the partner will acknowledge this gesture and respond with love. But instead of understanding the sacrifice, the partner may feel indebted or overwhelmed by the responsibility of maintaining a relationship that rests on a fragile emotional balance.

The Cycle of Sacrifice and Frustration

The cycle of sacrifice is a vicious circle in which the emotionally dependent person finds themselves trapped. Each time they annul themselves for the other, they hope for an emotional reward, a gesture that shows the sacrifice has been appreciated and recognized. But when this recognition doesn't come—and it rarely does as expected—the person enters a cycle of frustration and further sacrifice.They convince themselves they haven't done enough, that they need to sacrifice even more to earn the other's love. So, they give up even more of themselves, hoping that this time the sacrifice will be recognized. But the more they sacrifice, the more they lose touch with their own essence, and the harder it becomes to see the relationship for what it truly is: an imbalanced bond, where sacrifice never leads to satisfaction but only to growing suffering.This cycle can continue for years until the dependent person finds themselves completely emptied, devoid of identity, living a life that no longer belongs to them. Every small piece of themselves has been sacrificed on the altar of love, leaving behind a deep void, a sense of self-loss that is difficult to recover without a process of awareness and healing.

Awakening: Rediscovering Oneself

Breaking the cycle of personal sacrifice requires an inner awakening. The first step is to recognize that authentic love does not require self-annihilation. True love is based on reciprocity, on accepting the other, and on a relationship where both partners are free to be themselves without having to give up their identity.The path to healing involves a process of self-discovery, where the person begins reconnecting with their own needs, desires, and dreams. It is a difficult journey because it requires confronting the fear of abandonment and the belief that without sacrifice, the other will be lost. But in reality, it is through reclaiming one's autonomy and self-worth that a healthier relationship can be built, where love is no longer a currency of exchange but a free expression of affection and sharing.

Conclusion

Personal sacrifice is one of the clearest signs of emotional dependency and carries with it a process of self-annihilation that can slowly destroy a person's identity and happiness. One lives for the other, through the other, forgetting who they are, what they desire, and what their deepest needs are. Sacrifice becomes a form of control, a desperate attempt to maintain the relationship, but ultimately, it only leads to frustration, resentment, and suffering.Rediscovering oneself is the key to breaking this destructive cycle. Love cannot be authentic if it requires the annulment of self, and only by recognizing one's intrinsic value and learning to respect one's own needs can a relationship be built where both partners are free to exist as complete individuals and not merely reflections of each other. True love does not require the sacrifice of one's essence but is nurtured by mutual freedom and respect.

Dysfunctional Relationships: Accepting Emotional and Physical Abuse

Dysfunctional relationships are like poisoned gardens. On the surface, they may appear normal, even flourishing, but beneath, they hide rotten roots nourished by fear, pain, and submission. In these relationships, love becomes an illusion, and the bond between partners transforms into an emotional prison, where abuse—be it emotional, physical, or psychological—is accepted, tolerated, and even justified. The person trapped in a dysfunctional relationship finds themselves in a cycle of pain from which escape seems impossible, accepting actions and words that should be intolerable and sacrificing their dignity for the illusion of love that no longer exists.

The Subtle Descent into Abuse

Entering a dysfunctional relationship isn't always obvious. It often begins with small signs, seemingly harmless behaviors that, over time, evolve into toxic dynamics. Emotional abuse may initially disguise itself as overprotection or overwhelming jealousy, behaviors that can seem like signs of intense affection. The partner may say things like, "I do this because I love you so much" or "I can't stand the thought of losing you." Instead of seeing these as warning signs, they are often mistaken for expressions of passionate love.Gradually, these signs intensify. The partner's demands become more controlling, comments more demeaning, and the other's freedom increasingly limited. It starts with small criticisms: "You can't do anything right," "No one loves you like I do," "You're lucky to have me." Repeated over time, these phrases carve an invisible wound in the psyche, progressively eroding the person's self-esteem.As the emotional abuse becomes more apparent, the person involved may feel confused and isolated, unable to understand what is happening. The abuser alternates moments of affection with acts of psychological cruelty, creating emotional dependency: the victim begins to believe that, despite everything, the partner is the only one who could love or accept them. This cycle of pain and contempt followed by apparent reconciliation makes it even harder to distinguish true love from abuse.

Emotional Abuse: Invisible Scars

Emotional abuse is one of the earliest signs of a dysfunctional relationship but also one of the hardest to recognize. It leaves no visible marks, no bruises, but it carves deep scars in the soul. The emotionally abused person begins to lose their identity, their confidence, and their sense of self-worth. The abuser manipulates the other's feelings, making them constantly feel inadequate or guilty.Phrases like, "You're worthless," "Without me, you're nothing," "Do you realize how much you make me suffer?" are common in these dynamics. The abusive partner uses words as weapons, inflicting pain that, though invisible, can be devastating. The goal is not only to hurt but to control: the abusive partner seeks to create emotional dependence, where the other feels they cannot live without them.Isolation is another typical tool of emotional abuse. The abuser tries to separate the victim from the outside world, from friends, and from family, progressively reducing their support system. "They don't love you like I do," "They're turning you against me," "Can't you see they're just trying to drive us apart?"—phrases that push the victim to sever ties with those who could offer an outside perspective, leaving them alone with their tormentor.Gradually, the victim begins to doubt themselves, their perceptions of reality. The abuser may resort to manipulation techniques like gaslighting, making the victim believe their emotions and perceptions are invalid: "You always exaggerate," "You imagined that," "I never said that." This leads the abused person to question their own judgment, convincing themselves that the only way to maintain the relationship is by conforming entirely to the partner's will.

Physical Abuse: Violence That Breaks the Silence

When physical abuse surfaces in a relationship, it is often preceded by a long period of emotional and psychological abuse. Physical aggression doesn't arise out of nowhere; it is the culmination of a dynamic of power and control built over time. Sadly, many people end up justifying physical abuse, convinced that it was an isolated moment of anger or that they were somehow responsible.Physical abuse can take many forms: slaps, punches, shoving, or even less visible acts like restraining, dragging, or physically preventing the other from leaving a room during an argument. The body becomes the battleground on which the abuser asserts their power, a territory to control and dominate.The person subjected to this abuse often enters a spiral of fear and submission. Physical violence is not just an act of aggression; it is a message of dominance: "I can hurt you; I control your body, your freedom." Faced with this constant threat, the victim walks on eggshells, trying to avoid any behavior or word that might trigger the violence.Even after an act of violence, the abusive partner may try to manipulate the situation by asking for forgiveness, downplaying the incident, or even blaming the victim: "You made me angry," "I didn't mean to, but you provoked me." This cycle of violence and reconciliation becomes an even more effective control mechanism, as the victim, hoping the aggression won't happen again, accepts the apologies and convinces themselves that things might get better with time.

Justifying the Abuse: The Prison of Hope

One of the most complex aspects of dysfunctional relationships is the victim's ability to justify the abuse. Even when faced with unacceptable behaviors, many people continue to hope that their partner can change, that the pain is only temporary, that love will redeem the other. This hope is fueled by memories of happier times, promises of change, and the fear of being alone.The abused person may convince themselves that the abuser is not truly bad, that they are simply hurt or incapable of managing their emotions. "They're going through a rough time," "They're not always like this," "They love me but don't know how to show it"—these are common phrases in such dynamics. The victim tends to minimize the abuse, finding excuses that make acceptable what should never be accepted.But this justification is nothing more than an invisible prison. The victim, bound by hope and fear, cannot see that the abuse is not an isolated act but a dynamic rooted in power and control. The more the abuse is justified, the more the cycle of violence is perpetuated, as the abuser knows they can manipulate the situation, promising changes that will never come.

The Cycle of Violence: An Endless Spiral

Dysfunctional relationships often follow a well-defined cycle: a period of growing tension, followed by an explosion of violence, and then a phase of calm and reconciliation. During the tension phase, the victim senses something is wrong, that the partner is more irritable or distant, but they try to avoid conflict, walking on eggshells to maintain peace. However, this constant state of alert is unsustainable, and eventually, an explosion of violence occurs—emotional, physical, or psychological—where the abuser unleashes their anger and need for control.After the violent episode, a phase of apparent calm follows. The abuser may apologize, justify their behavior, or even promise to change. This offers the victim temporary relief and reignites hope that things might improve. But in reality, the calm is only temporary, and the cycle repeats, trapping the victim in a spiral of suffering that seems never-ending.

Liberation: Breaking the Cycle

Breaking free from a dysfunctional relationship is incredibly difficult. The victim, trapped between fear and hope, must confront not only the abusive partner but also their deepest fears: the fear of being alone, the fear of not being loved, the fear of not being enough.But liberation is possible. The first step is recognizing that abuse—whether emotional or physical—is never justifiable and that no one deserves to live in a relationship based on fear, control, or pain. Often, the support of friends, family, or professionals can be crucial in helping the victim see reality and find the courage to leave.

Conclusion

Dysfunctional relationships, marked by the acceptance of emotional and physical abuse, are traps that swallow dignity, self-esteem, and freedom. The victim becomes ensnared in a cycle of violence, hope, and reconciliation, unable to see that true love can never grow from fear or submission. Breaking these dynamics requires immense courage, but it is the only way to rediscover oneself, to free oneself from control and pain, and to rebuild a life based on authentic love, respect, and freedom.

Chapter 5: The Impact of Emotional Dependency on Daily Life

Effects on Mental Health: Anxiety, Depression, and Stress

Dysfunctional relationships, marked by toxic dynamics of control, manipulation, and abuse, do not merely cause emotional pain; they inflict deep wounds that can devastate the mental health of those involved. Anxiety, depression, and stress are not just occasional symptoms, but constant companions in these tumultuous relationships, draining every ounce of peace and trapping the mind in a cycle of fears, insecurities, and obsessive thoughts.Although these effects are invisible to the outside eye, they silently erode the inner self, creating a paralyzing reality that infiltrates every aspect of daily life. The mental and physical symptoms are the external manifestations of a deep discomfort, a cry for help from the soul that struggles to breathe under the weight of a dysfunctional relationship. Let's explore how these destructive forces manifest and transform the lives of those affected.

Anxiety: The Constant Sense of Danger

Anxiety is often the first sign of distress in a dysfunctional relationship. When a relationship is dominated by unpredictable dynamics, where love and aggression alternate chaotically, the mind can never find peace. Anxiety becomes a constant presence, an invisible thread that keeps the person in a state of hyper-vigilance. Every word, gesture, and silence from the partner can feel like a potential threat, triggering a continuous flow of worry.The person in a dysfunctional relationship is always walking on eggshells, trying to avoid anything that might trigger conflict or violence, whether emotional or physical. Even a simple unanswered message or a curt remark can provoke paralyzing anxiety. "What did they think?" "Why are they angry?" "What did I do wrong this time?" These thoughts play like a broken record in the mind, preventing the person from relaxing, enjoying peaceful moments, or focusing on other aspects of life.Anxiety seeps into every facet of daily life. It manifests in physical symptoms—tachycardia, trembling, muscle tension—and psychological ones—intrusive thoughts, an inability to concentrate, and constant worry. The person feels trapped in a constant state of emergency, as though something terrible could happen at any moment. Even when things seem calm, anxiety lurks in the background, ready to resurface at the slightest hint of danger.This emotional hyper-vigilance drains the person's energy, leaving them exhausted and incapable of finding peace. Anxiety not only erodes their ability to handle daily stress but also leads to a growing inability to trust their own perceptions and judgments, fueling a sense of helplessness and frustration.

Depression: The Soul's Void

If anxiety is the symptom of uncertainty and constant fear, depression is the result of prolonged exposure to pain that seems inescapable. The person in a dysfunctional relationship, constantly subjected to emotional, physical, or psychological abuse, begins to internalize the pain. Self-esteem gradually erodes, and over time, the person starts to feel devalued, useless, and incapable of escaping their situation.Depression seeps in like a heavy fog, smothering any joy or hope. Emotions fade, and what once brought pleasure or satisfaction becomes meaningless. The abused individual begins to doubt their own worth. The partner's cutting words, controlling behavior, and constant humiliations all contribute to an inner narrative in which the victim sees themselves as inadequate and unworthy of a better love. Their thoughts spiral into a vicious cycle: "Maybe they're right, I'm not enough," "Maybe I'm worthless," "I'll never be happy."This sense of powerlessness and despair leads to a slow descent into depression. Days blur into one another, feeling empty and purposeless. The person may feel disconnected from themselves and the world, unable to experience emotions—even negative ones. Depression isn't just sadness; it's the absence of emotion, an inner void that prevents the person from reacting or seeking escape.Chronic fatigue, difficulty concentrating, and loss of interest in daily activities are just some of the signs of depression. In dysfunctional relationships, the depressed individual feels trapped, unable to imagine a way out, convinced that suffering is an integral part of their existence. The mere thought of leaving the relationship may seem impossible, not just due to the fear of being alone but also because they believe there's nothing better out there for them.

Stress: The Erosion of Mind and Body

Stress is the common thread linking anxiety and depression in dysfunctional relationships. Living in a constant state of tension and fear has a devastating impact not only on mental health but also on physical health. Both the mind and body are subjected to unbearable pressure, leading to gradual deterioration that manifests in both physical and psychological symptoms.Chronic stress in a toxic relationship stems from the ongoing emotional tension, the need to anticipate the partner's reactions, and the constant effort to avoid conflict. The body responds to this tension with a series of physiological reactions: cortisol levels—the stress hormone—rise, the immune system weakens, and the body shifts into a constant survival mode.Symptoms of chronic stress may include headaches, gastrointestinal issues, insomnia, and a general sense of physical and mental fatigue. But stress doesn't only affect the body; the mind, continuously under unsustainable pressure, begins to falter. The person may feel overwhelmed, unable to handle even the smallest daily problems, and may overreact to situations that normally wouldn't cause concern.Constant emotional stress also leads to a loss of control over thoughts and emotions. The person may become easily irritated, lash out for no apparent reason, or, conversely, withdraw completely, unable to face any kind of confrontation. Stress is like a taut rope, ready to snap at the slightest touch, and in a dysfunctional relationship, that rope is constantly being pulled until it eventually frays.

The Downward Spiral: The Interconnection of Anxiety, Depression, and Stress

Anxiety, depression, and stress are not separate manifestations but feed into each other in a downward spiral. Anxiety, fueled by constant fear and emotional uncertainty, erodes mental and physical defenses, leaving the person exhausted and vulnerable. This vulnerability opens the door to depression, which takes hold when hope fades and the pain seems inevitable. Depression, in turn, intensifies stress, as living in a constant state of suffering increases the pressure on the body and mind, creating an endless cycle of pain.The result is emotional paralysis. The person feels trapped, unable to imagine a different life, lacking the strength or will to seek help. This downward spiral can last for years, leading to devastating consequences not only for mental health but also for physical health. Psychosomatic disorders, chronic illnesses, the deterioration of social relationships, and even the risk of developing addictions or self-destructive behaviors are all direct consequences of this destructive cycle.

The Path to Healing: Awareness and Courage

Breaking this cycle requires awareness and courage. The person trapped in a dysfunctional relationship must recognize the devastating impact the relationship is having on their mental and physical health and understand that they are not condemned to live in a constant state of suffering. But this recognition is only the first step. True change happens when they find the strength to seek help, to reach out for support, and to face their fears.Therapy can be a valuable tool in helping individuals understand the toxic dynamics of the relationship, recover their self-esteem, and learn how to manage anxiety, depression, and stress in healthy ways. Healing takes time, but it is possible. It is a journey of rediscovering oneself, rebuilding one's identity, and reclaiming inner strength.

Conclusion

Dysfunctional relationships inflict invisible but deep wounds on mental health. Anxiety, depression, and stress are just a few of the manifestations of a greater pain, a suffering that slowly corrodes one's ability to live peacefully and love oneself. However, recognizing these symptoms and understanding their connection to the dysfunctional relationship is the first step toward healing.Escaping this cycle of suffering requires an act of courage, an inner awakening that allows the person to see that they deserve more—that they deserve a life free from fear, depression, and stress. It is a difficult path, but in the end, it leads to rebirth: a return to freedom, serenity, and, most importantly, self-love.

Physical Effects: Insomnia, Eating Disorders, and Psychosomatic Illnesses

Dysfunctional relationships, burdened with emotional abuse, manipulation, and control, not only ravage the mind but leave deep scars on the body as well. The accumulated psychological pain, often repressed or unspoken, finds a way to manifest physically, as if the body itself were telling the story of the suffering the mind can no longer bear. Insomnia, eating disorders, and psychosomatic illnesses are some of the most evident manifestations of this inner torment, turning the experience of mental anguish into a cycle of physical pain. It is as if the body is crying out for attention and help, while the mind is too preoccupied with surviving the emotional prison of the toxic relationship.

Insomnia: Sleep Dissolved by Overthinking

Insomnia is one of the first physical signs that emerges in those living in a dysfunctional relationship. When the mind is trapped in a constant loop of anxiety, worry, and fear, sleep becomes an unreachable mirage. The bed, which should be a place of peace and rest, transforms into a battleground where thoughts crowd in, and the quiet of night amplifies every doubt and fear.People in toxic relationships often report feeling constantly on alert. Even when the partner is not physically present, the mind remains in a vigilant state, always ready to respond to a potential conflict, a cutting word, or abusive behavior. Thus, even when the body is supposed to relax and surrender to rest, the brain stays active, like an antenna constantly tuned to danger.Nights become long and tortured. Insomnia manifests in different forms: difficulty falling asleep, frequent nighttime awakenings, or the feeling of waking up exhausted, even after many hours of sleep. Thoughts of the partner, their unpredictable reactions, and unsaid words invade the mind in a relentless flow, allowing no respite.This lack of sleep not only mentally drains the person but also weakens the body. Without adequate rest, the immune system is compromised, making the person more vulnerable to illness and infection. Chronic fatigue also leads to diminished concentration, memory problems, and impaired decision-making, making it even harder to navigate the complexities of a dysfunctional relationship.Insomnia is not merely a lack of sleep but a lack of peace. It is the physical manifestation of a mind that cannot afford to rest, always ready to fight, always on the edge of a precipice.

Eating Disorders: The Body as a Battleground

Another physical effect that manifests in dysfunctional relationships is the emergence of eating disorders. When emotional pain becomes unbearable and anxiety consumes every thought, the relationship with food can turn into a means of control or self-punishment. The body becomes the battlefield for an invisible struggle between the desire to find comfort and the need to express pain that cannot find words.Some people, in response to emotional suffering, turn to food for comfort. Eating becomes a way to temporarily soothe anxiety and the inner void. Food provides immediate gratification, offering momentary relief from the constant pressure of the toxic relationship. However, this relief is only temporary and is soon replaced by guilt, self-disgust, and a sense of failure. Thus begins a cycle of binge eating followed by guilt, which only intensifies mental anguish.On the other hand, some people respond to emotional pain by restricting their food intake. The idea of controlling what they eat becomes a way to regain control over a life that seems to be slipping away. Skipping meals, reducing food intake, or following extreme diets can become a form of self-punishment, as if the body must pay for the inability to escape the dysfunctional relationship. In this case, hunger becomes a kind of penance, a way to punish oneself for not being strong enough or for failing to leave a toxic situation.Regardless of the direction the eating disorder takes, the impact on the body is devastating. Excessive weight gain or loss, digestive issues, nutritional deficiencies, and a decline in overall health are just some of the physical consequences of a dysfunctional relationship with food. But behind these physical manifestations lies emotional pain that cannot find another way to express itself except through the control and manipulation of the body.

Psychosomatic Illnesses: The Body Cries What the Mind Hides

Psychosomatic illnesses are the most complex and profound manifestation of the impact of a dysfunctional relationship on the body. In this case, emotional pain does not just disrupt sleep or affect eating habits; it transforms into real physical ailments. The body becomes a stage where the inner drama plays out through real symptoms: chronic pain, headaches, gastrointestinal problems, muscle tension, and autoimmune diseases.These symptoms, though lacking an immediately identifiable physical cause, are nonetheless real and debilitating. The body, unable to bear the weight of emotional pain any longer, transfers the discomfort to the physical realm. Psychosomatic illnesses represent a cry for help from the body, signaling that the mind is at its limit of endurance.A common example is chronic stomach pain, often linked to constant stress and anxiety. The person may begin suffering from ulcers, colitis, or gastritis—symptoms that may seem to have no clear cause but are, in reality, related to the emotional state. The body, constantly under tension, reacts with inflammation and disorders that mirror the internal distress.Headaches are another common sign of psychosomatic illness. Frequent headaches can result from accumulated tension, constant worry, and the repression of strong emotions like anger or fear. It's as if the mind can no longer contain the weight of these emotions and instead directs them to the body in the form of physical pain.In some individuals, the pain manifests even more complexly, through the development of autoimmune diseases. The immune system, weakened by emotional stress, may start attacking the body itself, leading to conditions like lupus, fibromyalgia, or rheumatoid arthritis. These diseases not only reflect the body's fragility in the face of emotional pain but also symbolize how the mind, under constant pressure, can turn inner suffering into physical illness.

The Body as a Reflection of the Mind

In a dysfunctional relationship, the body becomes the arena where the invisible battles of the mind and heart are fought. Every symptom, every physical ailment reflects the emotional pain the person is trying to suppress or manage. In many cases, the body speaks more clearly than the mind, showing through pain, fatigue, and illness what the person cannot express in words.Psychosomatic illnesses are a clear signal that emotional suffering has reached a level where it can no longer be ignored. The body, through its symptoms, seeks attention, signaling that there is a deep problem that needs to be addressed. Yet, in many dysfunctional relationships, these signals are ignored, minimized, or attributed to other causes, while the real root of the problem—the toxic relationship—continues to poison both mind and body.

Conclusion: The Body Cries for Help

Insomnia, eating disorders, and psychosomatic illnesses are just some of the physical manifestations of what happens inside a dysfunctional relationship. These symptoms are not only the result of emotional pain but are also signals that the body sends out as a cry for help, drawing attention to a suffering that can no longer be ignored.Breaking free from a toxic relationship is not just about escaping emotional or psychological abuse; it is also about reclaiming one's physical health, rebuilding a healthy relationship with the body, and restoring self-love. It is a healing process that takes time but ultimately leads to rebirth: a life where mind and body are no longer prisoners of pain but free to exist in harmony, finally free to breathe.

The Loss of Identity: When the Partner Becomes the Center of the Universe

There comes a moment, often invisible and silent, when love, which should enrich and expand our existence, begins to diminish, consume, and shrink our world into an ever-smaller dimension. This happens when the partner becomes the center of the universe, the axis around which every thought, action, and desire begins to orbit, leaving little or nothing for ourselves. It marks the beginning of the loss of identity, an insidious process where one gradually drifts away from their true self until they no longer recognize who they are.

In a healthy relationship, the partner is a life companion, an important part of our world, but not the entire universe. There is space for autonomy, personal dreams, and individual growth. But in dysfunctional relationships or when the bond becomes emotional dependency, the balance breaks, and the personal identity is gradually eroded until it vanishes, sacrificed on the altar of idealized love and the obsessive need to be loved.

The Dissolution Process: A Gradual Disappearance of Self

The loss of identity doesn't happen overnight. It is a gradual process, almost imperceptible at first, like a slow current that washes away pieces of ourselves, leaving behind a void that we try to fill with the other person's presence. We convince ourselves that this total fusion with the partner is a sign of deep love, a special and indissoluble bond. And so, we slowly begin to give up parts of ourselves, little by little.

It starts with everyday choices. Perhaps we stop seeing friends, give up hobbies, or spend less time on passions that once brought us joy. We justify these choices as necessary compromises to make the relationship work: "I'm doing it for love," "I don't want to upset him/her," "My free time is for him/her." But over time, these sacrifices become habits, and we find ourselves living solely for the other, without recognizing our inner voice.

Major life decisions begin to be made with the partner in mind. Life choices, career paths, and even ambitions are filtered through the lens of the relationship: "What will he/she think?" "Will I meet his/her expectations?" Every action is aimed at maintaining the balance of the relationship, and individuality is sacrificed to avoid conflict or ensure the other person stays close. We become increasingly dependent on their opinions, their approval, and we constantly adapt, until we lose touch with what we truly want.

Love as Self-Annulment

In a relationship of emotional dependency, love is no longer a feeling that enriches, but a force that consumes. The partner becomes a kind of savior, the only source of meaning and value. Without them, we feel lost, empty, and useless. We live in constant fear that, without that love, we will never be enough, never be whole. And so, we continue sacrificing parts of ourselves, hoping to keep the bond intact and avoid abandonment.

Self-annulment becomes a daily act. We conform to the tastes, habits, and desires of the other. We begin to speak their words, see the world through their eyes, and share their dreams as if they were our own. But in this process of fusion, we lose touch with our authenticity. We become a shadow of the other, a reflection of their inner world, and our own voice, thoughts, and desires fade away until they disappear completely.

Self-esteem is progressively eroded. We start depending entirely on the other for our sense of worth. If they are happy, we feel loved; if they are distant or angry, we feel inadequate, a failure. Our identity becomes defined by the partner's reactions, and our concept of self shrinks to a mere reflection of their emotions and judgments. This leads to extreme emotional fragility, where every gesture or word from the other can trigger waves of anxiety or despair.

The Eclipse of Passions and Dreams

The loss of identity is not just an emotional issue; it also involves personal desires and ambitions. Those who annul themselves for the other end up putting aside their dreams and aspirations, believing that the relationship is more important than any personal achievement. Careers, hobbies, friendships—everything is sacrificed in the name of love.

Dreams that were once vibrant and alive begin to fade, seen as superfluous or selfish. We stop pursuing goals that don't directly involve the partner, thinking that personal success might somehow jeopardize the balance of the relationship. Personal fulfillment is viewed as a threat, and we prefer to adapt, live in the shadows, content to exist only through the other's success or happiness.

In this state, life loses its color and depth. Every day is lived for the partner; every action is aimed at pleasing them or maintaining stability in the relationship. But in the process, we lose our passion for life, our ability to dream and desire beyond the relationship. We find ourselves living a life that no longer belongs to us, a life where we have abandoned our authenticity for a love that, instead of nourishing, consumes.

Emotional Dependency: When the Other Becomes Oxygen

The partner becomes the oxygen, the only reason to breathe. There is no more space for ourselves because our entire life revolves around them. The partner's presence becomes indispensable, and their absence unbearable. When they are near, there is relief; when they are distant, we live in a state of anxiety and terror. We become emotionally dependent, unable to face life alone, as if our existence no longer has value without the constant support and affection of the other.

This emotional dependency leads to an even deeper self-annulment. We stop having a life outside the relationship, losing touch with friends, family, and our inner world. All that matters is the partner. Every decision, every thought is aimed at keeping the relationship alive, and we live in constant fear that if the other were to leave, there would be nothing left to live for.

In this state, the individual loses all sense of autonomy. It becomes impossible to imagine an independent existence or even a happy life without the partner. Our happiness is entirely tied to the presence and mood of the other, and we live in a constant state of anxiety, trying to avoid any conflict or problem that might jeopardize the relationship. Our life becomes a reflection of the other, and we lose ourselves in the attempt to be what the other desires, forgetting who we really are.

Recognizing the Loss and Rediscovering the Self

Recognizing that we have lost our identity is an act of courage and awareness. It takes time to realize that love, instead of enriching, has drained us, and that our very being has been sacrificed to maintain a relationship that has stifled our authenticity. But this awareness is the first step toward healing.

Rediscovering oneself after living for the other requires a process of inner reconstruction. It is a painful journey, one that involves acknowledging our wounds, facing the fear of loneliness, and learning to know ourselves again. It means reconnecting with our desires and dreams and valuing them once more. It means accepting that true love does not require self-annulment, but demands respect and mutual freedom.

Conclusion: Finding One's Own Center Again

When the partner becomes the center of the universe, we lose ourselves in a fusion that leaves only emptiness and dependency. The loss of identity is one of the most devastating effects of dysfunctional relationships, as it strips the individual of their essence, turning love into an emotional prison.

But the path to freedom and rediscovery of self is possible. It means taking back control of one's life, learning to love oneself, and finding that inner center that was abandoned in the pursuit of the other. It is a journey of rebirth, where one rediscovers that happiness and self-worth do not depend on the other but on who we are, in all our authenticity.

The Effect on Other Relationships: Friendships, Family, and Work

When a dysfunctional relationship takes control of a person's life, the impact extends far beyond the intimate sphere between the partners. Like a shadow that slowly expands, this toxic relationship begins to invade every other aspect of life, devastating friendships, family relationships, and even professional life. Relationships that were once solid and sources of comfort become fragile, distant, drained by the constant tension and isolation that a toxic relationship inevitably brings.

In a healthy relationship, love is not an act of possession but an enrichment. The partner becomes an important part of one's existence, but not an obstacle to one's freedom. However, in dysfunctional relationships, a progressive closure to the outside world occurs. The partner becomes the center around which everything revolves, and other connections start to fade, as if there were no room left in the life of the person involved.

Isolation in Friendships: The Gradual Withdrawal

One of the most immediate effects of a dysfunctional relationship is the gradual withdrawal from friendships. Friendships, once a source of joy, support, and lightness, slowly become incompatible with the toxic relationship. Often, this distancing does not happen dramatically or abruptly, but through a series of small gestures, compromises, and renunciations, until one day the person realizes they are alone.

In a dysfunctional relationship, the partner may start to show jealousy or control over the other person's friendships. Comments such as, "I don't like you going out with them," "I'd rather we spend more time together," or "I don't understand why you need to see your friends so often" become common. At first, these might seem like small signs of possessiveness or requests for affection, but over time, they transform into subtle control. The person involved in the toxic relationship starts limiting their outings with friends, declining social invitations, hoping to avoid conflict or keep the peace with their partner.

As time passes, friendships cool down. Friends, feeling sidelined or seeing that the person is no longer present as they used to be, may start to distance themselves. This fuels a cycle of isolation, where the person trapped in the dysfunctional relationship loses external points of reference, cutting off the

people who could offer a different perspective or help them escape the toxic situation.

However, isolation is not always a personal choice: sometimes, the partner manipulates the situation, making the person feel guilty for every moment spent away from the relationship. Questions like, "Aren't I enough for you?" or "Why do you prefer spending time with them instead of me?" feed guilt and obligation, further pushing the person away from friends. Gradually, the shared laughter, confidences, and light-heartedness are replaced by a sense of loneliness and alienation.

The Fracture in Family Relationships: Distance and Conflict

If the withdrawal from friends is gradual, the effect of a dysfunctional relationship on family relationships can be just as devastating, if not more so. The family, which usually represents a safe haven and a place of unconditional support, becomes an emotional battleground where the toxic dynamics of the relationship spill over with intensity.

In many dysfunctional relationships, the partner attempts to isolate the person not only from friends but also from family. This can happen through psychological influence, with comments like, "They don't understand you like I do," "Your family is too intrusive," or "They don't care about our relationship." Gradually, the person starts to question their family, accepting that, to maintain peace in the relationship, they must reduce the time spent with them or even avoid certain family members.

This emotional distance from family can create painful fractures. Parents, siblings, or other relatives may begin to notice that something is wrong, that their loved one is changing, becoming more closed off, distant, and less available. However, attempts to intervene can lead to even more conflict. The person involved in the toxic relationship, defending their partner, may reject their family's help, seeing their concerns as an attack on the relationship or, worse, a betrayal.

Over time, family relationships cool or become a constant source of tension. Every family gathering becomes an occasion for conflict, with the family trying to make the person see that their partner is not a healthy presence, while the person clings even more to the relationship, hoping to prove everyone wrong.

This family isolation not only increases emotional dependence on the partner but also deprives the person of an important support system. Without the family's support, it becomes harder to find the strength to leave a toxic relationship, as the fear of being completely alone, with no one to rely on, intensifies.

The Deterioration of Professional Life: Stress and Distraction

Even professional life is not immune to the effects of a dysfunctional relationship. The emotional burden of constantly living under pressure, in fear of conflict or episodes of abuse, inevitably affects the workplace. The mental and emotional capacities needed to navigate daily professional life are severely compromised, and work, which once may have been a source of personal fulfillment, becomes an unsustainable burden.

The emotional stress caused by the relationship spills into the workday. The mind, always focused on the relationship, struggles to concentrate on professional tasks. Worries about the partner, unresolved conflicts, or the future of the relationship become obsessive thoughts that distract and reduce the ability to focus and be productive. One might find themselves staring blankly, unable to make decisions or complete even the simplest tasks because the mind is trapped in the toxic dynamics of the relationship.

In some cases, the dysfunctional partner may even interfere directly with professional life. There may be constant demands for attention, phone calls during work hours, or complaints about the time spent on work instead of the relationship. This creates internal tension, a sense of guilt for the time spent away from the partner, and the person may begin to neglect their career, sacrificing it in an attempt to keep the relationship intact.

Over time, the career may suffer severe consequences. Lack of focus, absenteeism, and decreased performance can lead to reduced opportunities for professional growth, conflicts with colleagues or superiors, and even real risks of losing the job. But again, the person trapped in the toxic relationship is often unable to see these signs as a warning because all their energy is focused on the relationship, which has become the sole center of their life.

Loneliness: A Growing Void

Ultimately, the most devastating effect that a dysfunctional relationship has on other relationships is the creation of profound and painful loneliness. The person, isolated from friends, distant from family, and alienated from their work, finds themselves alone, with the partner as the only point of reference. But this point of reference, instead of providing support and love, becomes a source of pain and control, amplifying the sense of emptiness.

This loneliness is particularly devastating because it is invisible. Those living in a toxic relationship often do not realize they are alone, believing that their partner's love is enough, that it is right to sacrifice everything to keep the relationship alive. But deep down, a sense of loss grows, a hidden awareness of having abandoned everything and everyone for something that no longer nourishes but consumes.

Conclusion: Rebuilding Connections and Rediscovering Oneself

Leaving a dysfunctional relationship does not just mean freeing oneself from the partner's control and manipulation; it also means rebuilding connections with the outside world. It means rediscovering the importance of friendships, family support, and finding pleasure and pride in one's work again. It is a process of rebirth, where one recovers not only their identity but also the sense of belonging to a network of healthy and enriching relationships.

True love never demands isolation or the sacrifice of everything for the other. On the contrary, healthy love expands, enriches all areas of life, and allows for the preservation of vibrant and intact relationships that make us complete as individuals.

Chapter 6: Emotional Dependence in Different Relationship Contexts

Romantic Relationships: Emotional Dependence in Love

Emotional dependence in romantic relationships is like a shadow that envelops love, an invisible yet powerful force that transforms what should be a free expression of affection into a suffocating bond, full of insecurities, fears, and unresolved needs. It is a love that, instead of nurturing, consumes; a love that, rather than enriching, demands continuous sacrifice, leading the dependent person to live not for themselves, but entirely through the other.

In a relationship dominated by emotional dependence, love becomes a golden cage in which the person trapped within fails to see the bars. There is a sense of completeness in the other, a visceral need for closeness that overwhelms and stifles, creating a bond not based on freedom but on a compulsive need for validation, reassurance, and constant presence. Love is confused with need, and emotional fusion is mistaken for a deep connection, when in reality, it is a form of self-annihilation.

The Illusion of Total Love: When the Other Becomes Everything

Romantic emotional dependence often stems from an idealized vision of love. One imagines that true love must be all-encompassing, a force that fills every inner void and gives meaning to every aspect of life. The partner becomes the reason for living, the sole source of happiness, the answer to every doubt and insecurity. Over time, the dependent person starts to see the other as the only one capable of understanding, supporting, and loving them unconditionally. In this process, they gradually lose their identity, becoming a reflection of the other.

The dependent person feels that, without their partner's love, their life would lose meaning. The other becomes the oxygen, the sun around which they orbit, and any distance, no matter how small, is experienced as an existential threat. Emotional fusion occurs, with boundaries between self and other dissolving, and the person begins to live only through their partner, as if their self-worth depended entirely on the partner's gaze, attention, and affection.

In this dynamic, love is no longer a reciprocal and free sentiment but an obsessive need. The dependent person constantly seeks the presence of the other, their approval, their affection, as if without it, they would be condemned to sink into an unbearable void. Every small act of separation—such as a missed call or a day without messages—can trigger a spiral of anxiety and anguish because the dependent person cannot conceive of life without the constant support of their partner.

Fear of Abandonment: The Dread of Being Alone

One of the most devastating aspects of romantic emotional dependence is the perpetual fear of abandonment. The dependent person lives in a state of constant insecurity, as if the bond is always on the verge of breaking, even without any apparent reason. Every sign, every silence, every shift in the partner's mood is perceived as a potential prelude to a breakup, generating unbearable anxiety.

This fear leads to obsessive behaviors. The dependent person constantly seeks reassurance, declarations of love, and gestures that prove the partner is still there, still in love, still committed to staying. The partner becomes an emotional anchor, and any moment of physical or emotional distance is seen as a threat to the dependent person's internal balance. In this dynamic, the dependent person becomes unable to live peacefully when the other is not near, developing a near-compulsive need to monitor the relationship, keeping it under constant scrutiny to prevent things from slipping out of control.

Jealousy is often a clear symptom of this fear of abandonment. Every interaction the partner has with others, every friendship, every external connection is viewed as a potential threat. The emotionally dependent person constantly fears being replaced, leading them to try to limit the partner's external relationships as much as possible. In some cases, this can result in obsessive control, where messages, social media, and outings are monitored—all in an attempt to keep the partner "under control."

Self-Sacrifice: Losing Oneself for the Other

One of the most profound and destructive effects of romantic emotional dependence is the self-sacrifice it entails. The dependent person not only lives for the other but also begins to progressively sacrifice every aspect of their life to please the partner. They give up their dreams, desires, and passions, convinced that by doing so, they can avoid conflict and keep the bond strong. Their life becomes a daily sacrifice, a constant adaptation to the other's needs and desires.

Over time, this self-abandonment leads to a deep loss of identity. The person no longer recognizes themselves, as every choice, decision, and action is made in function of the partner. They become incapable of asserting their own will, expressing their own desires, or saying "no" when necessary. Their inner world shrinks, flattens, and the sole objective becomes keeping the partner close, at any cost.

But this sacrifice never leads to happiness or balance. The more one gives up, the more suffocating the bond becomes, and the less room there is for genuine love. The partner, who initially seemed the center of the universe, progressively becomes a consuming presence, leaving only an unfillable void in their wake.

The Loss of Autonomy: Living Through the Other

Another critical aspect of romantic emotional dependence is the total loss of autonomy. The dependent person becomes incapable of doing anything without the support or presence of their partner. Everyday decisions, even the most trivial ones, must pass through the filter of the partner. They lose the ability to act independently, to make decisions on their own, to live their life autonomously.

In a healthy relationship, autonomy is a fundamental component. Each partner has their own space, interests, and emotional independence. But in emotional dependence, all of this vanishes. The dependent person lives in constant fear of upsetting or disappointing the other, so they conform as much as possible to their partner's expectations. They give up doing things they enjoy, abandon personal goals, all to avoid risking the loss of the relationship.

This lack of autonomy leads to extreme fragility. Without their partner, they feel lost, unable to face life on their own. Even minor daily challenges seem insurmountable because the dependent person has lost touch with their inner strength and ability to act independently. In this state, the partner becomes not just central but the only lifeline, the sole source of security, and any separation is experienced as catastrophic.

Breaking the Cycle: Rediscovering the Self

Breaking free from romantic emotional dependence is a long and painful process, but it is possible. The first step is recognizing that the relationship being lived is not a healthy love but a form of dependence. It requires facing one's fears, confronting the inner void, and learning to find within oneself what has always been sought in the other. Only through a process of self-awareness and rediscovery of personal value can the cycle of dependence be broken.

Therapy can be a valuable tool in this journey. With the help of a professional, one can begin to explore the deep roots of emotional dependence, often tied to past traumas, low self-esteem, or a deep-seated fear of abandonment. Learning to build healthy boundaries, regain autonomy, and cultivate self-love are the first steps toward a new life, one in which love is no longer a suffocating bond but a free and mutual choice.

Conclusion: Authentic Love is Freedom

Romantic emotional dependence is a distorted form of love, where need takes the place of desire and fear replaces trust. When the partner becomes the center of the universe, one loses their essence, sacrifices their identity, and love becomes a cage that imprisons rather than liberates.

But true love, real love, never asks for the sacrifice of oneself. Healthy love is a balance of closeness and distance, of sharing and autonomy. It is a bond where both partners can grow, realize themselves, and live their lives in full freedom—without fear, without obsessive need, but with the certainty that the relationship is based on mutual respect, trust, and the freedom to be fully oneself.

Chapter 6: Emotional Dependence in Different Relationship Contexts

Family: Dynamics of Dependence Between Parents and Children

The family is the first emotional refuge, the place where individuals develop their sense of belonging and identity. In this space, the relationship between parents and children should represent a balance of unconditional love, care, and support, allowing children to grow freely and independently, ready to face the world with confidence. However, this balance is not always achieved, and in some families, emotional dependence dynamics develop, where the boundaries between parents and children blur and confuse, transforming what could be a loving bond into an emotional prison that stifles the growth and freedom of both.

The dynamics of emotional dependence between parents and children manifest in different ways but share a common denominator: the inability to let the other be free. Whether it is the parent exercising excessive control over the children, or the children being unable to emotionally detach from the parents, the result is an unbalanced relationship where autonomy is sacrificed for a bond that, despite being filled with love, becomes suffocating.

The Parent's Dependence: Living Through the Child

In some families, emotional dependence originates with the parents, who, in their desire to maintain a close and unbreakable bond with their children, end up stifling their independence. This phenomenon is particularly evident when parents project their insecurities, fears, and unfulfilled desires onto their children, attempting to live through them the experiences they feel they never fully had.

The dependent parent may try to control every aspect of the child's life, from minor decisions to significant choices such as education, career, and even romantic relationships. This need for control doesn't stem from bad intentions but rather from the fear of losing the bond with the child and being left behind once the child becomes independent. The dependent parent, therefore, seeks to maintain constant, intrusive influence, often justifying this behavior with worry and excessive affection.

Phrases like "I'm doing this for your own good," "You don't know how much I worry about you," or "Without me, you wouldn't know what to do" are common in these dynamics. Behind these words lies a deeper desire: to keep the child close, preventing them from building an independent life. The dependent parent cannot imagine their life without a constant bond with the child, and every attempt by the child to distance themselves is experienced as rejection or abandonment.

Often, this dynamic leads the parent to project their unmet expectations onto the child. The child becomes the means through which the parent attempts to fill emotional voids or compensate for personal failures. As a result, the child's choices are continually judged, directed, and manipulated, with the hope that by following a predetermined path, they will become what the parent wanted to be. In this process, the child progressively loses touch with their own desires, living in an emotional shadow where it becomes impossible to distinguish between what they truly want and what the parent desires for them.

The Child's Dependence: Fear of Disappointing

Emotional dependence doesn't only develop from the parent's side. In many cases, children struggle to emotionally detach from their parents, living in constant fear of disappointing them or losing their affection. This type of dependence often manifests in children raised in environments where love was conditional upon compliance and obedience. From an early age, these children learn that to be loved, they must meet their parents' expectations and behave as desired.

Over time, this need for approval becomes emotional dependence. The child struggles to make decisions on their own, constantly fearing failure and judgment. Every choice is weighed against how it will be perceived by the parents, and the desire not to disappoint becomes the driving force behind all actions. This dynamic often leads to a life devoid of authenticity, where the child never develops a true sense of identity, perceiving themselves only as an extension of the family's expectations.

In extreme cases, the emotionally dependent child may forgo their dreams and desires to maintain their parents' love and approval. The fear of rejection or causing emotional conflict within the family becomes so overwhelming that it suppresses any attempts at independence. This creates an invisible prison where the child remains trapped, trying to become what the parents want, without ever being themselves.

The Cycle of Guilt: Emotion as a Tool for Control

One of the most powerful tools that fuels the dynamics of dependence between parents and children is guilt. The dependent parent, often unknowingly, uses guilt to keep the child emotionally tethered, preventing them from breaking free. Phrases like "After everything I've done for you, you're leaving me alone?" or "Don't you see how much I suffer?" or "You're all I have left" are subtle ways to make the child feel responsible for the parent's happiness.

This creates an emotional trap that is difficult to escape. The child, feeling guilty for the parent's pain, convinces themselves that it is their duty to stay close, to sacrifice their autonomy to prevent further suffering. In this way, guilt becomes a force that stifles any attempts at emancipation, keeping the child chained to a relationship of mutual dependence.

On the other hand, the dependent parent may use their emotional pain as leverage to get what they want. By appearing fragile or incapable of facing life without the child, the parent maintains control over them, wielding what seems to be a simple plea for affection but is actually a way to avoid confronting their own loneliness or insecurities.

The Consequences of Dependence: The Stunted Growth of Both Parties

The dynamics of dependence between parents and children have devastating consequences, not only for the children but also for the parents. On the one hand, children grow up lacking a sense of independent identity, unable to develop their own life and constantly living under the shadow of their parents. This lack of autonomy often leads to unfulfilled personal development, as the child continuously strives to meet external expectations without having the courage to pursue their own dreams or desires.

On the other hand, the parents suffer as well. Their emotional dependence on their children prevents them from building a life beyond the parental role. They fail to construct a new phase of life based on different relationships, personal interests, or fulfillment independent of their children. They remain trapped in the past, unable to evolve or face their own vulnerabilities.

This lack of mutual growth creates a static relationship where both parents and children remain stuck in roles they can't transcend. The parent can't see the child as an independent adult, and the child can't see themselves outside the family context. This emotional stagnation leads to latent frustration that may last for years, manifesting in unresolved conflicts, emotional tensions, and a constant sense of dissatisfaction.

Breaking Free: Ending the Cycle of Dependence

Breaking the cycle of emotional dependence between parents and children requires awareness on both sides. Parents need to learn how to let go, allowing their children to become independent, make mistakes, and lead autonomous lives—even if this means temporary distance. They must confront their own fears and insecurities, learning to build a life that is based on support rather than control.

Children, in turn, must recognize their own value independently of their parents' approval. They need the courage to pursue their own dreams, even if this means disappointing family expectations. Only then can they build an authentic life based on their desires, not those imposed from outside.

Conclusion: Love That Liberates

The dynamics of dependence between parents and children are among the most complex and painful, as they stem from a deep but misdirected love. However, true love, the kind that allows growth and fulfillment, is a love that liberates, not imprisons. It is a love that supports, that accepts autonomy, and that allows both parents and children to be themselves without fear or guilt, but with the understanding that the greatest love is one that empowers, not one that controls.

Toxic Friendships: When Affection Becomes a Trap

Friendship, in its purest form, is one of the most valuable bonds we can experience. It enriches life, offering support, joy, and understanding. However, not all friendships are born of this light. Sometimes, a connection that should nurture becomes a burden, an emotional trap that suffocates and consumes. In what we call toxic friendships, affection transforms into a power struggle, where one friend manipulates, controls, and emotionally drains the other, making them feel trapped in a relationship that is no longer free, but oppressive.

A toxic friendship is insidious. Often, it begins with the best intentions, with a strong bond based on shared experiences, deep affection, and emotional closeness. But over time, without us realizing it, this bond starts to change shape. We find ourselves caged in a relationship where affection is tainted by manipulation, jealousy, and the need for control.

The Disguised Beginning: False Complicity

Toxic friendships rarely present themselves as such from the start. In fact, they often begin with a deep sense of complicity. There's a feeling of harmony, of an elective affinity that seems almost unique. You share everything: thoughts, secrets, fears, dreams. It's like finding a person who finally understands every aspect of your life. In this initial phase, the toxic friend may appear as the most loyal and available person, someone who seems to have only your best interests at heart.

However, behind this apparent loyalty and devotion lies a darker desire: the need for possession. The relationship gradually becomes exclusive, and the victim of this toxic friendship may not immediately notice the shift. The toxic friend starts to demand to be the only confidant, the only point of reference. Every other friendship or relationship is seen as a threat. Slowly, the toxic friend begins to isolate the other, often using subtle manipulation tactics.

Phrases like: "I'm the only one who truly understands you" or "Others don't know you like I do" become tools to reinforce their position and sow doubt. The bond tightens, but in this increasingly constrictive embrace, the other's freedom begins to disappear. You find yourself trapped in a relationship where, every time you try to pull away, you are pulled back with guilt and demands for loyalty.

Emotional Manipulation: Affection and Guilt

One of the hallmarks of toxic friendships is emotional manipulation. The toxic friend uses affection as a tool to control the other, leveraging their feelings of loyalty and the desire to maintain the friendship. Every time the other tries to assert their independence or set boundaries, the manipulator responds with a mix of guilt and victimization.

If the toxic friend senses emotional or physical distance, they may respond with phrases like: "You're never there for me," "You're drifting away—what did I do wrong?" or, in more extreme cases, "You've changed, you're not the person I trusted anymore." These words serve a dual purpose: making the other feel guilty for needing space and recreating a bond of emotional dependency. The implicit message is that "Without you, I can't be okay."

This alternating between affection and guilt becomes an emotional trap. The toxic friend can make the other feel responsible for their emotional well-being, creating a relationship of dependence that becomes harder and harder to break. Every attempt to assert one's individuality is met with resistance, often accompanied by dramatic declarations of abandonment, leading the victim of the toxic friendship to give in, fearing to hurt or lose someone they care about.

Subtle Control: Jealousy and Isolation

In toxic friendships, control often takes subtle but dangerous forms. It frequently manifests as jealousy towards other friendships or relationships. The toxic friend does not want the other to have strong ties with other people, fearing they might lose their central role. This leads to progressive isolation.

Whenever the victim of the toxic friendship tries to spend time with others, the toxic friend may react with subtle jabs or passive-aggressive comments: "Oh, you're going out with them? I guess you don't have time for me anymore..." or "Did you have fun without me?" These remarks are not overtly aggressive but hide a clear manipulative intent. Their goal is to make the other feel guilty, to insinuate that their loyalty and dedication aren't enough.

Over time, the victim may start to avoid other friendships or limit their time with others to avoid negative reactions. The toxic friend thus succeeds in isolating the victim, maintaining total control over the bond. This dynamic becomes a prison: the more one submits to control, the more they drift away from others, and the fewer emotional resources they have to escape the toxic relationship.

The Exhaustion: When Friendship Becomes a Burden

One of the most devastating effects of a toxic friendship is the emotional exhaustion that results. Maintaining the bond with a toxic friend becomes increasingly draining because the relationship demands continuous effort, constant attention to the other's needs, and unceasing vigilance to avoid conflict or guilt. Every encounter, every conversation seems loaded with tension, as if something is always unresolved, something to worry about.

In a toxic friendship, there is no longer reciprocity. The relationship becomes one-sided, centered on the needs and insecurities of the toxic friend, while the other is forced to sacrifice their emotional well-being to keep the peace. You feel emptied, with no energy left for yourself, unable to receive the emotional support that, in a true friendship, should be present. Over time, the weight of this relationship becomes unbearable, but paradoxically, the more trapped you feel, the harder it becomes to leave, because the affection, though tainted, still holds a strong emotional grip.

Breaking the Chain: Liberation from a Toxic Friendship

Breaking free from a toxic friendship is a painful challenge because it involves acknowledging a reality you often prefer to ignore: that the bond is no longer healthy, that the affection has been corrupted by control, and that the friendship is no longer a source of joy but of suffering. This recognition is the first step towards liberation.

Breaking the chain requires courage and self-esteem. The victim of a toxic friendship must learn to set healthy boundaries and recognize that their emotional well-being cannot be sacrificed to please a manipulative friend. It is necessary to take a step back, reduce contact, and, if necessary, walk away from the relationship entirely. This detachment can be extremely difficult, especially because the toxic friend will often react dramatically, trying to leverage guilt and fear of abandonment.

But only through this process of detachment can you regain your freedom. It's a journey of emotional healing, where you learn to recognize your own needs, prioritize your well-being, and seek friendships based on reciprocity, respect, and support—not manipulation and control.

Conclusion: True Friendship is Freedom

Toxic friendships are bonds that imprison, turning affection into an invisible trap of guilt, control, and manipulation. Escaping these bonds is an act of courage and self-love. True friendship, the authentic kind, does not demand emotional sacrifices or impose limits on freedom. It is a bond that enriches, offering mutual support without asking for anything in return except the freedom to be yourself.

In a healthy friendship, there are no power plays, no impossible demands, no subtle manipulations. There is only the freedom to grow together, to share joys and sorrows without suffocating the other. When affection becomes a trap, it's time to break free, to shatter the chains, and seek a greater love: the love for oneself and one's own freedom.

Emotional Dependency in the Workplace

Emotional dependency, often associated with romantic or familial relationships, can also manifest in professional environments, where power dynamics and the need for approval intertwine subtly, creating an invisible trap for those involved. In a workplace where competence, autonomy, and responsibility should define relationships between colleagues, employees, and supervisors, emotional dependency can undermine not only individual performance but also emotional balance and mental health.

Emotional dependency at work is a psychological attachment where the individual constantly seeks the approval and affection of supervisors or colleagues, sacrificing their independence, self-esteem, and often dignity. This dependency extends beyond the need for professional validation and transforms into an emotional craving for recognition, exceeding the normal desire to be appreciated at work.

The Need for Approval: When Self-Esteem Depends on the Office

One of the key elements of emotional dependency at work is the obsessive need for approval. Instead of relying on solid self-confidence, the emotionally dependent person constantly seeks external validation to feel worthy. Every task, project, and interaction with superiors or colleagues becomes a test to prove their value.

This need for approval leads the individual to submit to the expectations and desires of others, progressively relinquishing their professional autonomy and independence. It's no longer about being a good worker but about pleasing superiors, adapting to their views, and ensuring there's never a reason for disappointment. The workplace shifts from being a space for professional growth to an emotional arena where the person desperately seeks to be loved and accepted.

However, the praise and recognition they receive provide only temporary relief. The emotionally dependent person struggles to derive lasting satisfaction from their achievements. No matter how much validation they receive, insecurity always lingers, ready to resurface at the slightest criticism or sign of disapproval. This creates an endless cycle of anxiety and stress, where negative feedback is amplified and experienced as an emotional catastrophe.

The Power Dynamic: Submission to Superiors

A distinctive aspect of emotional dependency in professional settings is the imbalanced relationship with superiors. The dependent person often develops a kind of obsessive admiration for their boss or manager, viewing them not only as an authority figure but also as an emotional mentor, someone whose judgment becomes indispensable for their sense of self-worth.

This type of relationship can lead to dangerous levels of emotional submission. The emotionally dependent individual rarely dares to contradict their superior, accepts any request—no matter how unjust or disproportionate—and goes above and beyond in hopes of gaining recognition or affection. They take on excessive workloads, work impossible hours, and are willing to sacrifice their personal time and well-being to maintain the superior's trust.

Often, the superior is unaware of how much the dependent person is sacrificing to please them. However, in some cases, these superiors may take advantage of the situation, exploiting the employee's need for approval to ensure unconditional submission. In this context, emotional dependency not only limits the person's professional growth but also strips them of dignity, making them incapable of defending their rights or asserting their needs.

Professional Jealousy: Competition and Fear of Rejection

Emotional dependency in the workplace can also breed professional jealousy toward colleagues. The dependent person constantly fears being replaced or losing the favor of superiors to a more competent, brilliant, or visible colleague. This can lead to unhealthy competitive dynamics, where the individual no longer works to improve or grow but to protect their fragile dependent relationship with superiors.

In this context, every colleague's success is perceived as a threat. A form of performance anxiety develops, making every workday a battle to maintain the trust and esteem of superiors. The emotionally dependent person struggles to collaborate healthily because every partnership feels like a competition, an opportunity to prove their worth compared to others.

This professional jealousy often leads to isolation. Unable to see colleagues as resources or partners, the person retreats inward, becoming more dependent on the exclusive relationship with their superiors. But in this isolation, they lose opportunities for growth, exchange, and learning, remaining trapped in a cycle of emotional dependency that stifles professional evolution.

The Sacrifice of Well-Being: Work as Life's Purpose

One of the most devastating consequences of emotional dependency in the workplace is the sacrifice of personal well-being. The emotionally dependent person cannot draw a line between professional and personal life. Work becomes their reason for living, and every other aspect of life—family, friends, leisure—is relegated to second place.

This leads to emotional and physical burnout. The person never allows themselves a break, never refuses an assignment, or takes time for themselves, fearing disappointing their superiors or losing the recognition they've earned. They agree to work overtime, always be available, sacrifice weekends, vacations, and even their health, hoping this will prove their worth and secure their emotional bond with superiors.

But this constant sacrifice comes at a high cost. Exhausted from work, the individual begins to suffer from chronic stress, anxiety, insomnia, and other health issues related to overwork. The mind is constantly occupied with work-related thoughts, worries about maintaining status, or avoiding mistakes. This not only compromises mental and physical well-being but also limits the ability to enjoy life outside the office.

The Awakening: Recognizing Dependency and Rediscovering Autonomy

Breaking the cycle of emotional dependency in the workplace requires deep inner work. The first step is recognizing that the need for approval and affection, while human, cannot become the foundation of a professional career. Building healthy self-esteem means learning to evaluate one's worth based on skills, effort, and results—not the judgment or affection of others.

Learning to set healthy boundaries is essential. This means recognizing that it's okay to say "no" to excessive demands, that it's permissible to have a life outside of work, and that personal well-being must always be a priority. This awareness also requires the courage to confront the fear of disappointing or being rejected and to accept that the approval of superiors is not an indicator of personal worth.

The journey toward recovery from emotional dependency at work can be long and challenging, but it also marks a personal rebirth. One rediscovers the ability to act autonomously, make independent decisions, and collaborate with others without feeling competitive. Most importantly, they learn that professional satisfaction comes from within, not from external approval.

Conclusion: Working to Grow, Not to Depend

Emotional dependency in the workplace is an invisible but powerful trap, capable of turning work from a place of growth and fulfillment into a space of emotional suffering. Breaking free requires courage, self-awareness, and the ability to reclaim autonomy.

Work should be an opportunity to develop skills, build healthy professional relationships, and contribute meaningfully. When one can break the bond of emotional dependency, work returns to being what it should be: a tool for growth, not an emotional prison. Only in this way can one build a career based not on the search for approval but on the genuine value they bring.

Attachment and Emotional Dependency

John Bowlby's Attachment Theory: Attachment Styles John Bowlby's attachment theory, a cornerstone of developmental psychology, provides a fundamental understanding of human relationships. Through his research, Bowlby observed that the emotional bonds formed in childhood, particularly between a child and their primary caregiver, have a lasting impact on how people experience relationships throughout life. His theory reveals that the love, support, and security we receive in our early years are not fleeting memories but deeply ingrained patterns that shape how we perceive love, closeness, and even separation.

According to Bowlby, these early bonds create internal working models that influence how we relate to others as adults. These models give rise to three primary attachment styles: **secure, anxious,** and **avoidant.** Each style reflects a different way of experiencing intimacy and emotional closeness, based on childhood experiences.

Secure Attachment: Trusting in Love and Being Loved

A **secure attachment** is the most balanced and healthy of the attachment styles. People who develop this style have had consistent care, unconditional affection, and emotional stability from their primary attachment figure (usually parents) during childhood. Children with secure attachment feel safe exploring the world, knowing they can rely on an adult to protect and nurture them. This basic trust, built over the years, becomes fertile ground for healthy and fulfilling future relationships.

In adulthood, those with a secure attachment style tend to approach intimate relationships with calmness and trust. They are capable of giving and receiving love without fear of rejection or abandonment. These individuals can express their feelings honestly and authentically, without the need to manipulate or control the other person. Secure attachment allows for a relationship based on reciprocity, where each partner can support the other in difficult times without losing their own identity.

Securely attached people can also tolerate temporary separation from their partner, knowing that love and affection are not threatened by physical or emotional distance. They do not live in constant anxiety about being abandoned because they have internalized the belief that their worth does not depend solely on the approval of others. This emotional stability enables them to build lasting relationships where trust is the central pillar.

Anxious Attachment: Love as an Obsessive Need

Anxious attachment develops when a child receives inconsistent or unreliable care from their primary attachment figure. Sometimes the caregiver is present and attentive, while at other times, they are distant or unavailable. This alternation between closeness and absence creates deep insecurity in the child. Not knowing for sure when they will receive the love and affection they need, the child learns to live in anxiety, constantly seeking the caregiver's presence to feel safe.

In adulthood, this translates into relationships characterized by a constant fear of abandonment. People with anxious attachment tend to experience love as an obsessive need. They have an insatiable desire for reassurance and often interpret any sign of emotional distance as an impending rejection. Every silence or pause in communication can trigger a wave of anxiety and worry. These individuals crave constant closeness and may become jealous, possessive, or overly attached to their partner.

Their anxious attachment style leads them to experience relationships as an emotional rollercoaster. When they feel loved and close to their partner, they experience intense euphoria, but this feeling can quickly fade in the face of a small sign of distance. Love is lived with intensity and drama, and the partner may feel suffocated by the constant demand for attention.

The fear of abandonment pushes them to sacrifice their own needs or to overly adapt to please their partner in the hope of maintaining stability in the relationship. However, this behavior can lead to frustration, as no matter how hard they try, they never feel truly secure in the love they receive. Emotional instability and emotional dependency are typical traits of this attachment style.

Avoidant Attachment: Distance as Protection

Avoidant attachment develops when a child, from an early age, perceives that their emotional needs are not met or understood by their attachment figures. Parents of avoidant children may be distant, cold, or emotionally unavailable, creating in the child the idea that affection and emotional closeness are not things they can count on. Faced with this reality, the child learns to emotionally distance themselves to protect against the pain of rejection. The message they internalize is that relying on others is dangerous and that it is better not to count on anyone.

In adulthood, people with avoidant attachment tend to maintain emotional distance in their relationships. They may appear self-sufficient, independent, or even detached. While they may desire love and intimacy, they fear vulnerability and emotional dependence. This leads them to avoid deep emotional involvement, as they try to protect themselves from potential disappointment.

Avoidantly attached individuals struggle to express their feelings and manage emotional intimacy. They may withdraw when their partner tries to get too close because they perceive emotional closeness as a threat. In relationships, they may appear cold or indifferent and often prefer to focus on practical

or superficial aspects rather than addressing emotional issues. However, this does not mean they do not experience deep emotions but that they have learned to suppress them to avoid facing vulnerability.

This dynamic leads to relationships where the partner may feel neglected or unloved, while the avoidant individual may feel suffocated by the partner's emotional demands. Consequently, they may maintain emotional distance even in close relationships, viewing intimacy as a threat to their independence.

Conclusion: The Roots of Love and Fear

Bowlby's attachment theory provides a valuable lens through which we can understand how we love and relate to others. **Secure, anxious, and avoidant attachment styles** are deeply rooted in early childhood experiences and shape how we perceive love, trust, and intimacy throughout our lives. These styles are not fixed, and with time, awareness, and experience, it is possible to alter how we love, learning to manage fears and build healthier, more fulfilling relationships.

Secure attachment represents the ideal, a foundation of trust and reciprocity from which stable and rewarding relationships can grow. However, even those with anxious or avoidant attachment styles can work on themselves to overcome their fears and insecurities. The ability to love authentically, freely, and consciously comes from self-awareness, the willingness to face one's vulnerabilities, and the understanding that intimacy is not a threat but a source of enrichment.

The Influence of Childhood Attachment on Adult Relationships

Every human carries within them, like a silent echo, the experiences of their childhood. The early years of life are a crucial period where the deepest emotional bonds are formed, and these initial connections between a child and their attachment figures—usually parents—shape how that person will experience relationships for the rest of their life. It's as if, through these primary bonds, we learn to write our "vocabulary of love," which will accompany and influence every future relationship, especially romantic and intimate ones.

John Bowlby's attachment theory teaches us that how we were loved and cared for as children has a lasting impact on how we will love and be loved as adults. The attachment styles we develop in childhood—secure, anxious, or avoidant—become the filters through which we perceive love, trust, and intimacy in adult relationships. In other words, the emotional experiences of our childhood, often imprinted on our unconscious, largely determine our ability to build healthy, balanced relationships or, conversely, relationships filled with tension, fear, and insecurity.

Secure Attachment: The Serenity of Loving and Being Loved

Those who have experienced secure attachment in childhood enjoyed a stable and loving emotional presence from their parents or caregivers. The child felt accepted, protected, and learned that the world of affection is a safe place where they can trust others. This bond of trust creates a solid foundation that, in adulthood, manifests in the ability to live relationships with calmness and openness.

Adults with a **secure attachment** style can express their feelings without fear of being judged or rejected. In their relationships, they seek and offer intimacy, support, and emotional closeness. They have internalized the concept that love is not a battle to be won, but a place of reciprocity. This allows them to tolerate difficulties and conflicts without viewing every disagreement as a threat to the entire relationship.

A person with secure attachment does not fear temporary separation because they know that love does not dissolve with distance. They do not constantly seek validation, as they have already internalized their worth, independent of their partner's approval. This enables them to build relationships based on trust and collaboration, where both partners can grow and realize themselves individually without feeling constrained by the emotional bond.

Anxious Attachment: The Fear of Losing and Being Abandoned

The emotional fate is different for those who developed **anxious attachment** during childhood. These children experienced inconsistent affection: sometimes their parents were present and attentive, other times they were distant or inaccessible. This created deep insecurity, a sense of never being completely sure of the love and protection they needed. Over time, this translates into a constant anxiety about separation and the fear of being abandoned.

In adulthood, these individuals tend to approach relationships with anxiety and worry. They have a deep, obsessive need for emotional and physical closeness, fearing that any small distance or silence might precede abandonment. As a result, they can be jealous, possessive, and in need of constant reassurance. It's not that they don't love, but their fear of not being enough or losing the love of the other drives them to control, suffocate, and constantly seek validation.

Adults with an anxious attachment style are often on an emotional rollercoaster: when they feel close to their partner, they experience an intense sense of security and happiness, but even a small sign of distance or disinterest can send them into anxiety and doubt. This creates a dynamic of emotional dependency, where the person is willing to sacrifice their own needs and desires to maintain the relationship.

Avoidant Attachment: Escaping Intimacy

People with an **avoidant attachment** style learned during childhood that their emotional needs were not met. Their parents were often distant, unavailable, or incapable of responding to the child's emotional needs. Faced with this lack, the child developed a form of emotional self-protection: they learned to rely only on themselves and not expect anything from others.

In adulthood, this translates into difficulty with intimacy. Avoidantly attached individuals fear vulnerability and struggle to express their feelings. While they desire emotional relationships, they tend to avoid deep emotional involvement, maintaining a certain distance to protect themselves. They may appear indifferent, cold, or even insensitive, not because they don't feel emotions, but because they've learned to suppress them to avoid being hurt.

Avoidant adults struggle to handle their partner's emotional needs and often interpret closeness as a threat to their independence. When they feel too involved, they tend to withdraw, close themselves off, or find excuses to maintain emotional distance. This creates relationships that lack true intimacy, where the partner may feel neglected or unloved, while the avoidant individual fights to maintain control over their emotions and avoid becoming too attached.

The Attachment Cycle: When Styles Meet

Adult relationships often involve a meeting of different attachment styles, which can lead to complex and sometimes painful dynamics. For example, an **anxious** partner may find themselves in a relationship with an **avoidant** person, creating a sort of emotional dance where one partner chases while the other flees. The anxious partner, constantly seeking closeness, may make the avoidant feel suffocated, pushing them further away. In turn, the avoidant partner's emotional withdrawal only amplifies the anxious partner's fears of abandonment. This kind of dynamic can be difficult to break, as both partners react to their own fears, triggering a cycle that reinforces insecurity and distance.

However, it's important to note that attachment styles are not fixed. With awareness, therapy, and experience, people can modify their attachment style, learning to better manage their insecurities and build healthier, more satisfying relationships.

Healing Through Conscious Love

The journey to transform anxious or avoidant attachment styles requires deep self-awareness and an understanding of one's relational dynamics. Learning to recognize one's defense mechanisms, which may have originated in childhood, is the first step toward change. Those with an anxious attachment style can work on developing greater self-confidence, learning that it's unnecessary to control or constantly seek reassurance to feel loved. Likewise, those with an avoidant style can learn to allow themselves to be vulnerable, understanding that intimacy is not a threat to their independence but a source of mutual growth.

Adult romantic relationships offer a great opportunity for healing. Through conscious love, individuals can rewrite their internal attachment models. A loving, understanding partner can help break the cycle of fear and insecurity by providing a safe space where both partners can explore their vulnerabilities and learn to trust each other.

Conclusion: Childhood as a Root and a Starting Point

The influence of childhood attachment on adult relationships is profound and enduring. The emotional experiences of the early years shape how we see love, trust, and intimacy, creating patterns that we often unconsciously repeat in our adult relationships. However, these dynamics are not immutable. With awareness, openness, and a willingness to face our fears, it is possible to transform childhood wounds into opportunities for growth and to build healthier, more authentic, and fulfilling relationships.

In the end, every love story, every bond, offers the chance to rediscover ourselves, heal from our insecurities, and learn that true love is not born of fear but of trust.

Insecure Attachment and Emotional Dependency

Love is one of the most powerful and mysterious forces that guide our lives. When we love and feel loved, we experience a sense of security and wholeness that allows us to face the world with courage and confidence. However, not all experiences of love are free and fulfilling. For many people, love becomes a source of anxiety, fear, and above all, **emotional dependency**. This dependency often stems from the deep roots of **insecure attachment**, an emotional bond formed in childhood that influences how we experience relationships in adulthood.

According to **John Bowlby's attachment theory**, insecure attachment develops when, as children, we did not receive stable, consistent, and unconditional affection. Parents or caregivers were not always emotionally or physically available, creating fertile ground for insecurity. The child, who relies entirely on adults for their well-being, cannot develop a secure base from which to explore the world. This uncertainty becomes internalized and later manifests as a profound fear of being abandoned, rejected, or unloved. This internal model of relationships is carried forward as an emotional inheritance into adult relationships, giving rise to what we call **emotional dependency.**

The Roots of Insecure Attachment: The Fear of Not Being Enough

Insecure attachment can develop in various ways, but it always stems from a sense of inadequacy and the constant fear of losing love. Children who grow up in environments where affection is given inconsistently—sometimes present, other times distant or even absent—learn to live in a continuous state of needing reassurance. They never know for sure when or if they will receive the love they need. This creates a constant sense of alertness, a desperate need for closeness and attention to feel safe.

In adulthood, this experience turns into a constant need for validation in relationships. People with insecure attachment often interpret love not as a feeling of peace and serenity but as a battle to maintain their partner's closeness, as if every moment of emotional distance is a threat to the entire bond. They live in fear that their partner may suddenly pull away, stop loving them, or even abandon them. This generates a cycle of fear, possessiveness, and control that ultimately traps both individuals in a suffocating relationship.

Emotional dependency is essentially the adult version of that **childhood need for security and reassurance.** In relationships, those with insecure attachment tend to **idealize their partner,** attributing them with an almost salvific power. The partner becomes not just a person with whom to share life but an emotional lifeline, the only one capable of giving meaning and value to their existence. The relationship thus becomes a **prison of affection,** where love is no longer a free choice but a necessity.

The Cycle of Emotional Dependency: Love and Fear Intertwined

People with insecure attachment tend to experience love with dramatic intensity. Every gesture, every word, every silence from the partner is scrutinized and interpreted, often exaggerated, as a signal of closeness or, conversely, a possible abandonment. Emotional dependency is fueled by a deep-rooted fear of being left alone, and this fear pushes the individual to constantly seek reassurance and validation, sometimes even at the cost of sacrificing their dignity or personal needs.

In a relationship marked by emotional dependency, love is experienced as an emotional rollercoaster. When the partner is present and affectionate, the dependent person feels euphoria and relief. But as soon as they perceive a sign of distance—even the smallest—their mind is flooded with panic. A storm of intrusive thoughts arises: "Do they still love me?", "What did I do wrong?", "Why do they seem distant?" These thoughts fuel a compulsive need for control, which can lead to obsessive behaviors such as monitoring the partner, seeking constant validation, or even creating emotional drama to get attention.

In this dynamic, **love becomes a struggle not to be abandoned**, and the dependent person constantly lives in fear. Every sign of distance is experienced as a deep wound, and even when the partner reassures them, the relief is only temporary. As soon as the reassurance is given, the fear of losing it resurfaces. This creates an endless cycle of anxiety and dependency, where the need for emotional security becomes the sole driving force of the relationship.

The Sacrifice of Self: Losing One's Identity for the Sake of Love

One of the most painful effects of emotional dependency is the progressive **loss of identity**. The dependent person, in a desperate attempt to maintain the relationship, begins to sacrifice parts of themselves. Their own dreams, desires, passions, and even opinions are set aside in the hope that by pleasing the partner, they can avoid the feared abandonment.

Those with insecure attachment tend to conform to the other person's expectations, even when these conflict with their own needs. They stop asking for what they need, expressing their emotions, or setting healthy boundaries. The dependent person becomes a mirror of the partner, trying to mold themselves into what they believe will please or satisfy them. But in this process, they lose touch with their own authenticity and sense of self.

This **self-suppression** inevitably leads to a sense of emptiness and frustration. Even if the relationship continues, there is no longer room for individual growth or authentic self-expression. The dependent person lives in the shadow of their partner, in a relationship that, while seeming solid, is actually fragile and unbalanced. Emotional dependency suffocates the individual, creating a relationship based on need rather than mutual, free love.

The Illusion of Control: Trying to Govern Love

Another hallmark of emotional dependency, stemming from insecure attachment, is the **illusion of control**. The dependent person believes they can maintain the stability of the relationship through emotional control, attempting to influence the partner's behavior with constant demands for attention, love, and reassurance. However, **love is not something that can be controlled or governed**. It is fluid, ever-changing, and trying to force or hold onto it only worsens the situation.

In this context, the attempt to control often manifests as **jealousy and possessiveness**. The dependent person constantly fears that someone else might take their place, that their partner might find a new source of affection and support. This leads to behaviors of monitoring, unfounded suspicions, and a constant need to verify the partner's loyalty and dedication. But the more one tries to control love, the more it slips away, generating a cycle of insecurity and tension that undermines the stability of the relationship.

The Path to Healing: Recognizing and Breaking the Cycle

Breaking the cycle of emotional dependency requires **awareness and inner work**. The first step is recognizing that the need for control and constant validation is not a sign of love but of deep insecurity. The individual must begin to explore their fears, asking themselves where this sense of never being enough comes from and why they experience love as a battleground rather than a safe haven.

It is essential to **reclaim one's identity**. Instead of constantly seeking to please the other, the dependent person must rediscover who they truly are, what their needs, desires, and limits are. This requires a process of **self-acceptance and self-care**, where the person learns to value themselves independently of others' judgment or approval.

Therapy can be a great help in this process, providing a safe space to explore one's emotional dynamics, understand the roots of insecure attachment, and work towards developing a more secure attachment style. Learning to tolerate separation, manage anxiety, and build authentic trust in relationships is a crucial step in freeing oneself from emotional dependency.

Conclusion: The Freedom to Love Without Chains

Insecure attachment and emotional dependency are like **invisible chains** that bind love to fear. Those trapped in this dynamic live constantly on edge, in a desperate search for affection and reassurance that, paradoxically, ends up driving away the very love they desire. However, it is possible to break these chains. Through awareness, healing, and self-discovery, love can once again become what it is meant to be: **free, mutual, and fulfilling,** a safe place where both partners can grow together without fear of losing or being abandoned.

The Evolution of Attachment Style Over Time

Attachment styles, formed in early life in response to the care and love we receive, are not fixed or unchangeable. Just as people grow and evolve, so too can their approach to relationships and love. Attachment, like all aspects of the human psyche, is a dynamic process influenced by our experiences, interactions, and choices throughout life. What may begin as an insecure bond, full of anxiety, fear, or avoidance, can gradually transform into a healthier and more fulfilling way of relating, given the right self-awareness and effort.

This evolution results from inner growth, fueled by the willingness to confront our fears, break free from old emotional patterns, and learn to engage with love and intimacy in a healthier, more conscious way. The experiences we live through—whether in romantic relationships, friendships, or even our work and self-relationship—can become opportunities to reshape our attachment style. Though the journey can be long and difficult, it is filled with potential for transformation and healing.

The Influence of Relationships: Healing Through Love

One of the most powerful forces that can influence the evolution of attachment style is relational experience. Adult romantic relationships act as a mirror, reflecting our attachment patterns, highlighting the dynamics we unconsciously repeat, and offering a way out of toxic patterns.

For example, a person with an **anxious-insecure attachment** style, who lives with constant fear of being abandoned or unloved, may find a partner with a **secure attachment** style capable of offering unconditional love and emotional stability. In such a relationship, the anxious individual can slowly learn to trust and realize that love is not threatened by every moment of silence or temporary distance. Through this experience, they can begin to build more self-confidence and manage anxiety in healthier ways without constantly seeking reassurance.

Similarly, someone with an **avoidant attachment** style, who tends to flee intimacy out of fear of vulnerability, may be "challenged" by a partner who is patient and willing to offer a safe space to explore feelings. Over time, this individual may start to discover that closeness is not a threat to independence but rather an opportunity for mutual growth. Love becomes less about control or defense and more about sharing experiences.

Thus, **mature and conscious love** has the potential to heal attachment wounds. Stable, healthy relationships based on mutual respect provide fertile ground for transforming insecure attachment styles, helping individuals develop new ways of experiencing intimacy and trust. However, it's essential for both partners to be willing to engage in this growth process, recognizing their fears and insecurities and working together to overcome them.

Self-Awareness: The Key to Transformation

Another crucial factor in the evolution of attachment style is **self-awareness**. Modern psychology teaches us that recognizing our behavioral and emotional patterns is the first step toward change. Many people, upon discovering their attachment style, feel a sense of revelation, as if they finally understand the reasons behind behaviors or emotional reactions that seemed inexplicable up to that point.

This self-awareness is the starting point for transformation. When we begin to see how our attachment models influence the way we love, we can start working to change these patterns. For example, someone who identifies with an anxious attachment style can learn to manage their anxiety without constantly seeking external validation. Through practices of inner reflection and emotional work, they can develop a stronger sense of security within themselves, learning to meet their emotional needs independently.

Therapy can be a valuable aid in this growth journey. A therapist can help identify dysfunctional attachment patterns and guide a person toward developing healthier relationships. Through cognitive-behavioral therapy, couples therapy, or other forms of psychological support, individuals can learn to recognize their fears of abandonment or rejection and find more effective ways of managing these emotions.

Life Experiences: Evolution Through Pain and Resilience

Life experiences, particularly those involving pain and loss, can also profoundly impact the evolution of attachment style. Difficulties, disappointments, and even relationship breakdowns can become moments of personal growth. Although these experiences can be painful, they often force people to confront their vulnerabilities, bringing their attachment patterns into focus.

For instance, someone who has experienced a painful breakup may initially feel overwhelmed by fear of abandonment and loneliness. However, over time, this same experience can become an opportunity to learn how to be alone and to discover that love does not have to come exclusively from external sources. By learning to care for oneself, a person can develop greater emotional resilience, which can help transform an insecure attachment style into a more secure one.

These experiences aren't limited to romantic relationships but extend to friendships, family connections, and even how we face challenges in the workplace. Every time we experience loss, conflict, or rejection, we can choose to use these moments to reflect and grow. Over time, these difficult moments can help us develop a sense of self-trust that goes beyond the need for external validation.

The Power of Forgiveness: Letting Go of the Past to Embrace the Future

Another important step in the evolution of attachment style is **forgiveness**. People who have developed an insecure attachment often carry deep wounds linked to childhood experiences. Distant, inconsistent, or emotionally unavailable parents can leave emotional scars that affect future relationships. However, continuing to carry the weight of these wounds can prevent change and growth.

Forgiveness does not mean forgetting or excusing what happened, but rather learning to release the pain and anger to build a new way of relating. Forgiving the past—whether it involves a parent's behavior or one's actions in previous relationships—allows us to break the cycle of insecure attachment. Through forgiveness, we open the door to new emotional freedom, enabling us to embrace the future with more lightness and trust.

Conclusion: The Journey of Attachment Toward Freedom

The evolution of attachment style is a journey, not a destination. It is a process of discovery, self-awareness, and transformation that requires patience, commitment, and a deep openness to change. Even those who have lived with insecure attachment can, through the right experiences and conscious inner work, develop a more secure attachment and experience love in a freer, more authentic way.

Relationships, love, and even pain are milestones on this journey. While attachment style may be rooted in our early childhood experiences, our capacity to transform it and create new models of love and trust is limitless. Love, in all its forms, is a powerful tool for emotional healing and evolution, and every person has the potential to grow, change, and embrace deeper, more secure, and freer relationships.

The Role of Self-Esteem

Self-Esteem as the Foundation for Healthy Relationships

Self-esteem is like a hidden root, an invisible element that nourishes our worldview, how we relate to others, and, most importantly, the quality of our relationships. It is the secret core of every bond we form, the foundation upon which we build our ability to love and be loved. When this root is strong and well-nurtured, relationships grow to be healthy, balanced, and fulfilling. But when self-esteem is fragile or broken, relationships become complicated, suffocating, or even destructive.

Self-esteem, in essence, is the way we see ourselves: how deserving we feel of love, respect, and happiness. It is the internal voice that tells us whether we are worthy of being treated with kindness and consideration or if we should settle for less. It is not just a matter of ego but a deep inner belief about our own worth. And this belief influences every aspect of our relational life, determining the quality of the connections we make and how we behave within them.

Self-Esteem as an Emotional Compass: Recognizing One's Needs and Limits

Self-esteem is an inner compass that helps us navigate our behaviors and decisions, especially in relationships. When we have healthy self-esteem, we can recognize our needs and express them without fear. We aren't afraid to say what we want or ask for what we deserve because we know we are worthy of love, respect, and consideration. This allows us to build relationships based on true reciprocity, where both people can give and receive without sacrificing themselves.

A person with good self-esteem can set healthy boundaries and respect the boundaries of others. They don't feel the need to lose themselves or conform to be accepted because they already have solid confidence in their worth. Instead of creating distance, these boundaries protect and nourish the relationship, allowing both people to grow individually without losing themselves in each other.

On the contrary, those with fragile self-esteem tend to doubt their own worth. This doubt manifests in relationships as insecurity and emotional dependency. The person clings to the other, constantly seeking approval and validation to fill that inner void. But love, in this context, becomes more of an obsession than a free choice. The fear of rejection or abandonment pushes them to compromise their own needs, accepting situations where balance and reciprocity are absent.

The Freedom to Be Oneself: Authenticity and Trust in Relationships

Solid self-esteem gives us the freedom to be authentic in our relationships. When someone has confidence in themselves, they don't feel the need to wear masks or constantly adapt to what the other wants. Love doesn't become a continuous performance or an attempt to impress; instead, it becomes an encounter between two people who show themselves for who they are, with all their strengths and flaws.

Authenticity is the core of a healthy relationship. Without it, any bond is destined to be superficial and fragile. The ability to show one's vulnerabilities, insecurities, and imperfections is only possible when there is a deep acceptance of oneself. This acceptance creates a safe space where the other person can do the same, fostering a relationship built on mutual trust.

In a healthy relationship, both people know they don't need to be perfect to be worthy of love. They understand that the essence of love lies in accepting and embracing the other as they are, without trying to change or manipulate them. But this acceptance of the other cannot occur without first developing acceptance of oneself. Loving oneself is the first step in truly loving someone else.

The Risk of Self-Annullment: When Self-Esteem Is Fragile

When self-esteem is weak or damaged, relationships can become a breeding ground for insecurity and constant fear. A person with low self-esteem often thinks they are not worthy of the other's love, leading them to live in fear of abandonment or rejection. This fear creates a vicious cycle in which they try to please the other at all costs, often losing sight of their own needs and desires.

Those with fragile self-esteem may constantly worry they aren't good enough—whether attractive, interesting, or intelligent enough. This fear fuels a pattern of personal sacrifice, where they are willing to do anything to maintain the relationship, even at the expense of their own identity. The person stops being themselves, adapting to the partner's desires and expectations in the hope of not being left alone.

But this self-annullment never leads to happiness or relational stability. Instead, it fosters a toxic dynamic where one person sacrifices while the other, often unknowingly, takes, without realizing the harm being done. In a relationship where one person loses themselves, there is no room for true reciprocity. Love, instead of being a dance between two individuals, becomes a power play where one continually gives in and the other assumes control.

Personal Growth as a Pillar of Relationships

Healthy self-esteem not only positively influences relationships but also becomes the driving force behind personal growth within them. The most fulfilling relationships are those in which both people are committed not only to taking care of each other but also to growing together. This growth requires both individuals to have basic confidence in themselves, a belief that they are worthy of love and respect, and the ability to nurture their own dreams and aspirations within the relationship.

Self-esteem allows us to face challenges and difficulties in a relationship without falling into emotional drama or mutual dependency. When both people have confidence in themselves, they are capable of resolving conflicts constructively without seeing every disagreement as a threat to the relationship. Differences in opinion become opportunities for enrichment, not reasons for division.

Moreover, personal growth nurtured by solid self-esteem helps keep the relationship alive over time. When each partner continues to evolve, discover new aspects of themselves, and pursue their own dreams, the relationship becomes a space of continuous exchange. There is no stasis or stagnation, only a constant movement toward deeper, more mature love.

Conclusion: Love as a Reflection of Self-Esteem

Self-esteem is the invisible foundation upon which we build our relationships. Without it, love risks turning into dependency, fear, or self-sacrifice. With solid self-esteem, however, we can experience love in a free and conscious way, recognizing our own worth and allowing the other to do the same.

Healthy relationships are not born from the illusion of completing one another but from the certainty that each partner is already complete in themselves. Love becomes an encounter between two people who know their worth, who respect each other, and who choose to walk together not out of need but out of desire. This free choice, fueled by trust in oneself and in the other, is the foundation of every lasting and fulfilling relationship.

How Low Self-Esteem Fuels Emotional Dependency

Low self-esteem is a subtle and silent force that creeps into the most intimate corners of our lives, shaping how we see ourselves and the value we place on our experiences. When our self-esteem is fragile, we not only doubt our ability to be loved but also convince ourselves that the love of another is the only possible source of validation and recognition. In this dynamic, emotional dependency is born and grows, becoming a suffocating bond in which the person can no longer distinguish between love and need, between intimacy and emotional submission.

Emotional dependency feeds on an insatiable thirst for validation, a constant search for reassurance that stems from an inner void—a void we are unable to fill on our own. Instead of finding our value within ourselves, we desperately seek it from others, believing that only through their approval and affection can we feel complete. Low self-esteem, therefore, becomes the fertile ground on which emotional dependency grows and develops, turning love into a form of emotional imprisonment.

The Inner Void: The Lack of Self-Confidence

At the root of emotional dependency lies a deep inner void. Low self-esteem makes us believe that we are not worthy enough of love and attention, driving us to constantly seek validation from external sources. We live in constant fear of not being enough—enough to be loved, enough to be interesting, enough to be desired. Every relationship becomes a test of our worth, where we measure our importance based on how much the other loves or appreciates us.

Those who suffer from low self-esteem have a distorted view of themselves. Even when they receive affection and love, they often cannot internalize it. There is always a persistent doubt that corrodes them from within, an insecurity that makes them believe the other's love is fragile and could disappear at any moment. This creates emotional dependency, where the partner becomes an essential source of validation: without them, the person feels lost, empty, and unable to find meaning in their existence.

Low self-esteem makes us see every relationship as a kind of lifeline. Instead of believing we can be loved for who we are, we feel we must earn love, gain it through submission or sacrifice. This belief pushes us to idealize the partner, attributing to them an almost magical power to give us what we feel we lack—worth, security, identity.

The Need for Validation: The Hunger for Reassurance

Low self-esteem generates an insatiable hunger for reassurance. Those who don't believe in their own worth need to constantly feel loved, desired, and appreciated because they are incapable of finding these answers within themselves. This need for validation translates into emotional dependency, where the partner becomes the only source of well-being and security.

Every small sign of emotional or physical distance is perceived as a threat. If the partner isn't present enough, doesn't respond immediately to a message, or seems distracted, the person with low self-esteem falls prey to anxiety and panic. The dominant thought is: "They don't love me anymore," "They're going to leave me," or "I'm not enough for them." This fear fuels a cycle of obsessive behavior and jealousy, where they try to control the partner, hold onto them, and ensure they don't leave.

The need for validation can lead to manipulative or self-sacrificing behavior. The person with low self-esteem may stifle their own needs just to maintain the relationship. They become willing to do anything to please the other, even at the cost of losing their own identity and dignity. In this context, love becomes a form of emotional survival—a way to soothe the fear of not being enough, rather than a mutual choice between two people who want to share life together.

The Fear of Abandonment: The Terror of Loneliness

Another fundamental aspect of emotional dependency, fueled by low self-esteem, is the fear of abandonment. Those who don't believe in their own worth live in constant fear that the partner might leave them, abandoning them to face their inner void alone. This fear creates continuous tension in the relationship, turning love into a battle to avoid being abandoned.

The fear of abandonment drives the person to behave possessively or excessively dependently. There's a constant worry that someone else might take their place or that the partner might find a reason to leave. This leads to obsessive control over the relationship, where every gesture, word, or glance is interpreted as a sign of withdrawal or disinterest. The relationship becomes an emotional prison, where both partners are trapped in a dynamic of control and dependency.

This perpetual anxiety not only makes the relationship unstable but also prevents the person with low self-esteem from truly enjoying the love they receive. Every moment of joy is overshadowed by the fear that it might end. Every declaration of love is accompanied by the thought that it might not last. This distorted view of love, fueled by the fear of abandonment, makes it impossible to experience a genuine and fulfilling relationship.

Self-Sacrifice: Losing One's Identity to Maintain the Relationship

Low self-esteem not only creates emotional dependency but also leads to self-sacrifice. Those who lack confidence in their own worth are willing to do anything to maintain the relationship, even at the cost of losing their identity. This self-sacrifice manifests in compromising one's own needs, desires, and opinions to conform to the partner's expectations.

The person with low self-esteem often feels they don't deserve to be loved for who they are, so they try to change themselves to meet the partner's expectations. In this process, they lose their passions, interests, and even dreams. The relationship becomes a space where the only concern is keeping the partner close, even if it means completely surrendering their own will.

This self-annullment not only destroys the possibility of a balanced relationship but also generates resentment and frustration. In the attempt to please the other, the person distances themselves further and further from who they really are, ending up feeling empty and dissatisfied. The relationship, instead of being a source of mutual fulfillment and growth, becomes a cycle of dependency and sacrifice, where one person completely loses themselves.

Healing: Rebuilding Self-Esteem to Break Free from Dependency

Breaking the cycle of emotional dependency requires deep inner transformation. The key to freeing oneself from emotional dependency lies in rebuilding self-esteem. When a person learns to recognize their own worth, they realize that they don't need to depend on the love of others to feel complete. The first step is learning to give themselves love and recognizing that their happiness doesn't depend on someone else but on their ability to accept themselves with all their imperfections.

Therapy can be a valuable tool for exploring the roots of low self-esteem and working toward building a healthier self-image. Through psychological support, individuals can learn to recognize their own needs, establish healthy boundaries, and live relationships in a more balanced way without sacrificing their identity.

The healing process also requires facing the fear of loneliness. Only by learning to be okay alone, without emotionally depending on someone else, can one build a healthy and lasting relationship. When a person finds security within themselves, love becomes a conscious choice, not a desperate need for validation.

Conclusion: Love as a Choice, Not a Need

Low self-esteem is the fuel that drives emotional dependency, turning love into a continuous search for approval and security. However, authentic love is born from freedom and reciprocity, not from fear or the need to fill an inner void.

When we learn to believe in ourselves and recognize our worth, love no longer becomes a prison but a conscious choice. Instead of seeking validation from others, we find our security within, and we are able to build relationships based on mutual acceptance and respect. Only then can we truly love—not because we need to, but because we choose to, free from fear and dependency.

Strategies for Improving Self-Esteem and Achieving Emotional Independence

Self-esteem is the pillar upon which our sense of identity is built, an inner treasure that allows us to navigate life with confidence, resilience, and dignity. However, for many, this pillar is fragile, shaped by years of doubts, insecurities, and external conditioning. When self-esteem is low, we find ourselves at the mercy of events, other people's opinions, and especially relationships that end up defining our worth. From this condition arises emotional dependency, a state in which love, affection, and attention from others become essential for our emotional survival.

But there is a way out. Improving self-esteem and achieving emotional independence is an inner journey, a process of rediscovering your own value that requires time, patience, and commitment. It's not an immediate transformation but a gradual blossoming of awareness, confidence, and self-respect. The strategies below are designed to guide anyone willing to undertake this journey, to break free from the chains of insecurity and build a life where love, affection, and relationships are no longer a cage, but a free and conscious choice.

1. Cultivate Self-Awareness: The First Step Toward Independence

The first step in improving self-esteem is becoming aware of your thoughts, emotions, and the dynamics that lead you to doubt yourself. Often, low self-esteem results from deep-seated beliefs we've internalized over the years—distorted ideas about who we are, what we deserve, and what others expect from us. These beliefs are like inner voices that speak to us critically, judgmentally, and devaluingly.

Self-awareness is the ability to observe these voices without fully identifying with them. It allows us to distinguish between who we truly are and what we've learned to believe about ourselves. This process of observation takes time and attention, but it's crucial for breaking the cycle of low self-esteem.

- **Reflection exercise**: Keep a journal where you write every time you feel insecure or critical of yourself. Try to identify the moments when your self-esteem wavers and note the thoughts that arise. This will help you recognize your negative mental patterns and begin the transformation process.

2. Recognize Your Intrinsic Value: Love Yourself Unconditionally

Often, our sense of self-worth is tied to external factors—professional success, others' approval, physical appearance, or romantic relationships. But these factors are volatile and can easily change. To achieve solid self-esteem and emotional independence, we must learn to recognize our intrinsic worth, a value that doesn't depend on what we do or how we appear, but on the simple fact that we exist.

Loving yourself unconditionally means learning to accept your flaws, imperfections, and vulnerabilities, knowing that these don't make you any less deserving of love and respect. It is an act of self-compassion that allows you to treat yourself with the same kindness and understanding you offer others.

- **Self-compassion exercise**: Every day, take time to recognize something positive about yourself, even if it's small. Write a list of your qualities, achievements, or simply moments when you showed courage or kindness. Gradually cultivating a positive view of yourself is essential for improving self-esteem.

3. Learn to Set Healthy Boundaries: Protect Your Emotional Space

Low self-esteem often leads us to sacrifice our needs and please others for fear of rejection or abandonment. But to achieve emotional independence, we must learn to set healthy boundaries. This means recognizing that we have the right to say "no," to express what we desire, and to protect our emotional space.

Boundaries aren't walls, but guidelines that define what we're willing to tolerate and what we're not. They are a tool for maintaining balance in relationships, allowing us to be authentic and respect our needs without feeling guilty.

- **Boundaries exercise**: Identify a situation where you feel you didn't respect your emotional boundaries. Write down how you wish you had reacted, what you would have liked to say or do to protect yourself. This exercise helps you become more aware of your limits and practice assertiveness.

4. Develop Emotional Independence: Fill Your Inner Void

Emotional independence is the ability to manage your emotions without relying on others' approval or love to feel complete. It doesn't mean closing yourself off from others, but being able to find security and comfort within yourself, even when external circumstances don't provide it.

To develop emotional independence, it's important to learn to be alone without feeling lonely. This means cultivating your own company, finding joy and fulfillment in your passions, and building a life that has meaning and value, regardless of who is by your side.

- **Positive solitude exercise**: Set aside time each week to do something you enjoy, alone. Whether it's taking a walk, reading a book, or practicing a hobby, train yourself to enjoy your own company. This will help you develop emotional autonomy and discover that you can be happy without depending on others.

5. Accept Vulnerability: The Strength of Being Authentic

One of the biggest obstacles to self-esteem and emotional independence is the fear of being vulnerable. We often think that showing our weaknesses or needs makes us less worthy, and we try to hide these aspects of ourselves from others. But vulnerability isn't a sign of weakness—it's the courage to show yourself as you are, with all your imperfections, and accept that you can be loved for it.

Being authentic means allowing yourself to be truly seen, without masks. This authenticity requires courage, but it's also what allows us to build genuine relationships based on mutual acceptance.

- **Authenticity exercise**: The next time you feel the temptation to hide an emotion or a need out of fear of judgment, try expressing yourself honestly. Say what you feel without fearing how the other person will react. You'll discover that being vulnerable doesn't destroy relationships but strengthens them.

6. Recognize Successes and Celebrate Victories: Nurture Your Sense of Self-Esteem

Finally, one of the most important aspects of improving self-esteem is learning to recognize and celebrate your successes, even the small ones. Those with low self-esteem often focus on failures, minimizing their accomplishments. But it's crucial to learn to see your value and build self-confidence by celebrating your personal and professional victories.

- **Celebration exercise:** Every evening before going to bed, take a moment to think of three things you did well during the day. They can be small or big, but the important thing is to learn to recognize and appreciate your successes.

Conclusion: The Journey Toward Self-Esteem and Emotional Independence

Improving self-esteem and achieving emotional independence is a journey—a process that takes time, patience, and, above all, self-love. There's no magic formula, nor a final destination: it's a continuous process of rediscovery, where we learn, step by step, to free ourselves from the conditioning that has led us to doubt our worth.

Self-esteem isn't something given to us externally but an inner strength we can cultivate and nurture through self-awareness, self-compassion, and self-care. And when we learn to recognize our worth, respect our needs, and find security within ourselves, we become free to live healthier, more fulfilling relationships based on choice, not dependency.

The Path to Emotional Autonomy: Asserting Yourself Without Losing Yourself

Emotional autonomy is a valuable goal—a state in which an individual can maintain their inner integrity within relationships without losing themselves. It's the ability to be present for others without feeling diminished, to love without becoming dependent, and to assert your needs without compromising them for fear of losing the other person's affection. But the journey toward emotional autonomy is also complex, filled with challenges and discoveries, small steps leading to a deeper understanding of who we are and what we desire—without needing to find our identity reflected in someone else's eyes.

This path requires strength, awareness, and constant attention to the subtle difference between asserting and dominating, between loving and depending, between being autonomous and closing yourself off. Asserting yourself without losing yourself means finding a balance between the need to love and the desire to be free, between the wish for closeness and the necessity of protecting your emotional space. It's not a rigid or final condition but a delicate dance in which you learn to flow—sometimes failing, sometimes succeeding—in creating harmony between yourself and the world around you.

Emotional Autonomy as the Root of Inner Freedom

The first step toward emotional autonomy is recognizing that our emotional well-being should not depend entirely on others. From childhood, we are accustomed to seeking comfort and security in our caregivers—parents, friends, partners—and often learn to measure our worth by the love and approval we receive. This leads us to seek validation from others, as if we are incomplete without them.

But emotional autonomy stems from recognizing that we are already complete within ourselves. It doesn't mean living in isolation or depriving ourselves of relationships; rather, it's about learning to find our inner security, our center, without constantly relying on others' affection or attention. It's a freedom born from self-acceptance, rooted deeply within us, and not dependent on external validation.

Achieving emotional autonomy means developing the ability to be alone without feeling lonely, to feel content with ourselves, and not to desperately seek in others the key to our happiness. Only when we learn to recognize and value our uniqueness can we engage with others without turning into their reflection, without losing our essence.

Asserting Your Needs: The Courage to Say "I"

An essential element of emotional autonomy is the ability to assert your own needs. Many people, especially those with low self-esteem or a history of emotional dependency, find it difficult to express their desires and needs out of fear of rejection or judgment. They live in silent sacrifice, always putting others' needs first and neglecting their own in the hope of being accepted or loved.

But true love—whether for yourself or others—cannot exist without the ability to say "I." Asserting your needs isn't selfish; it's an act of self-respect. It's the courage to recognize that your desires, emotions, and aspirations are just as important as others'. Only when we learn to say "I" can we genuinely say "we," because a balanced relationship consists of two complete individuals, not a fusion where one person sacrifices themselves for the other.

- **Assertion exercise**: Every time you find yourself sacrificing a need to please someone, pause and reflect. Ask yourself, "What do I want in this situation?" and try to express your point of view clearly and assertively. Learn to say "no" when necessary, without fearing conflict. This is the first step in establishing a healthy balance between your needs and others'.

Setting Healthy Boundaries: Protecting Your Autonomy

To assert yourself without losing yourself, it's essential to learn to set healthy boundaries in relationships. Boundaries aren't walls that separate us from others but spaces of mutual respect that allow us to remain true to ourselves while engaging with others. They are the tangible expression of our personal value, the way we communicate to others where we end and they begin.

Those who struggle to set boundaries often find themselves in relationships where they feel overwhelmed or manipulated, unable to say "no" or protect their emotional space. This lack of boundaries leads to a gradual loss of identity, a sense of suffocation where you constantly feel obligated to meet others' expectations.

Setting boundaries means learning to defend your inner space without feeling guilty. It means knowing when it's right to be available and when it's necessary to retreat, without seeing this choice as a lack of love. When we manage to set clear boundaries, we protect ourselves from emotional erasure and can love authentically, without fear of losing ourselves in the other person.

- **Boundary exercise**: Whenever you feel overwhelmed or that you've sacrificed too much, take a moment to reflect on what you could have done differently. Write down a list of situations where you feel overrun or exploited and identify the boundaries you would have liked to set. This will help you recognize your limits and apply them in future interactions.

Inner Dialogue: Cultivating a Loving Relationship with Yourself

Emotional autonomy requires a healthy inner dialogue, one filled with self-compassion and kindness toward yourself. Often, our insecurity stems from a toxic inner dialogue—a voice inside that criticizes, judges, and makes us feel unworthy. This inner saboteur is the result of years of negative conditioning, but it can be reshaped through a conscious effort to rewrite our personal narrative.

Learning to speak to ourselves with love and understanding is essential for building solid self-esteem, and thus for asserting ourselves in relationships without fear of abandonment or rejection. When we are at peace with ourselves, we are less vulnerable to criticism and less dependent on external approval. Instead of desperately trying to conform to others' expectations, we feel secure in who we are, and this allows us to engage in relationships from a place of strength and authenticity.

- **Self-compassion exercise**: Every time you catch yourself being self-critical, replace that thought with an act of kindness. Imagine talking to yourself as you would to a dear friend going through a hard time. This will help you transform your inner dialogue from judgmental to compassionate, creating a space of love and acceptance within yourself.

The Power of Vulnerability: Asserting Yourself Without Defenses

Many believe that emotional autonomy implies a form of invulnerability, a detachment from others to protect oneself from pain. But in reality, emotional autonomy isn't about building walls—it's about remaining open and vulnerable without losing your integrity. Being emotionally autonomous doesn't mean being immune to pain or difficulties, but being able to experience them without being overwhelmed.

Vulnerability is an essential part of authentic relationships. When we're willing to show our vulnerability, we demonstrate a deep trust in ourselves and the relationship we're building. Vulnerability isn't weakness, but an act of courage, because it allows us to say, "This is who I am, with all my imperfections, and I choose to be open, even though I know I could get hurt."

- **Vulnerability exercise**: In your relationships, try expressing your deepest feelings without fear of being judged or rejected. Be honest about your fears, desires, and insecurities. This will help you build more authentic relationships and cultivate mutual trust.

Conclusion: The Path to Sustainable Emotional Freedom

The journey toward emotional autonomy is a path of balance, where you learn to assert yourself without losing yourself, to maintain your identity while remaining open to love and connection with others. It's not a goal reached once and for all, but a continuous practice—made of inner listening, self-compassion, and respect for your own needs.

Learning to be emotionally autonomous doesn't mean living without bonds, but creating relationships where the "we" doesn't stifle the "I," where love and reciprocity are conscious choices, not obligations or dependencies. When we learn to walk this fine line, we discover a new form of freedom—one that allows us to be truly ourselves without fear of losing who we are in the heart of love.

Chapter 9: Fear of Loneliness and Emotional Emptiness

Fear of Loneliness as the Driver of Emotional Dependence

The fear of loneliness is a shadow that silently creeps into our hearts, an invisible but powerful force guiding many of our choices, often without us being fully aware of it. This is an ancient fear, rooted in the human desire for belonging and connection, a condition that dates back to childhood when the closeness of others represented safety, protection, and love. However, when this fear becomes the primary engine of our relationships, it can turn into an emotional prison, fueling emotional dependence.

Emotional dependence is a condition where love is no longer a meeting of two free individuals, but an emotional necessity rooted in the fear of being alone. In this state, the other person is no longer simply a companion or someone to share life with, but a kind of lifeline, a refuge from the inner emptiness that loneliness makes us fear. The relationship thus becomes a shelter from our own shadow, and in order to avoid confronting the silence and emptiness we perceive within ourselves, we are willing to sacrifice everything—our freedom, our needs, and ultimately, our identity.

Inner Emptiness: Loneliness as an Existential Threat

At the core of the fear of loneliness often lies a deep inner emptiness, a feeling of incompleteness that makes us believe we are not enough on our own. This belief leads us to seek in others what we feel we lack within ourselves: love, security, and validation of our worth. In this context, loneliness is not just the absence of company, but a true existential void that we avoid at all costs.

Those who live with the fear of loneliness tend to develop a distorted view of relationships, seeing them as a kind of lifeline. The presence of the other becomes a shield against the feeling of emptiness, a way to fill the silence that frightens us. Instead of seeing the relationship as an encounter between two complete individuals, it becomes something to cling to, preventing us from being swept away by our sense of inner disorientation.

This fear is often fueled by low self-esteem and deep insecurity. When we do not believe we are worthy of love or capable of finding happiness on our own, we begin to see loneliness as a kind of punishment or a confirmation of our worst fears. This leads us to constantly seek external validation, believing that only through others can we find a sense of completeness.

Emotional Dependence: The Obsessive Need for Presence

The fear of loneliness generates an obsessive need for the presence of others. In romantic relationships, those who fear being alone desperately try to keep their partner close, even at the cost of sacrificing their own needs or accepting imbalanced and painful situations. Every sign of distance—an unanswered call, a delayed text, or a weekend spent apart—is experienced as a threat, a prelude to abandonment. Thus, emotional dependence develops, making it impossible to experience love freely and reciprocally.

People who fear loneliness often become jealous, possessive, and develop a constant need for reassurance. The partner becomes the sole source of emotional security, and every gesture or word is interpreted as either confirmation or threat to the relationship. The dependent person tries to control the relationship, holding on to it tightly, as if letting it flow naturally might make it slip away. In this attempt to hold on to the other person, the relationship loses its spontaneity and becomes an emotional prison, where love is replaced by fear.

Those who suffer from emotional dependence often find it difficult to be alone, even for short periods. Loneliness is experienced as an unbearable void, a time when their sense of insignificance grows stronger. Rather than seeing solitude as an opportunity for reflection, growth, and self-nourishment, it is feared as an absence of meaning, an emotional desert with no shelter.

The Sacrifice of Self: Losing Oneself for the Other

One of the most devastating effects of emotional dependence, driven by the fear of loneliness, is self-sacrifice. A person who fears being alone is willing to forgo their desires, set aside their needs, and even compromise their values in order to maintain the relationship. The presence of the other becomes so crucial that every disagreement or conflict is seen as an insurmountable threat, and any compromise is preferable to the dreaded solitude.

Those who live with the fear of loneliness tend to idealize their partner, attributing to them an almost salvific power. In this dynamic, the partner is not seen as an equal individual with whom to share life but as a source of life itself, without which they are doomed to sink into the void. This creates unbalanced relationships, where one person completely erases themselves, sacrificing their individuality, dreams, and ambitions to keep the other close.

But in this process of self-erasure, one gradually loses touch with themselves. The person no longer knows who they are outside the relationship, unable to imagine a life where the other is not present. In this way, love becomes a form of emotional imprisonment. The fear of loneliness turns love into a trap, where the connection with the other is seen as the only means of survival.

The Cycle of Fear: Loneliness and Mutual Dependence

The fear of loneliness can trigger a cycle of mutual dependence. In a relationship, both people often end up feeding this dynamic: one is afraid of being left alone, and the other feels compelled to meet that need, not out of authentic love but out of fear of hurting or being abandoned in return. This cycle creates a relationship in which neither person is truly free: one is bound by the anxiety of losing the other, while the other feels responsible for the partner's emotional well-being.

In this kind of dynamic, loneliness is never confronted, only avoided. The relationship becomes a continuous attempt to flee from oneself, to hide one's inner emptiness through the presence of the other. But this escape never leads to peace or lasting happiness, because true balance in relationships cannot be achieved when one's emotional foundation is built on fear and insecurity.

Facing Loneliness: The Path to Healing

Overcoming emotional dependence fueled by the fear of loneliness requires a courageous inner act: confronting one's loneliness without fear, learning to live with it, and most importantly, transforming it into an opportunity for growth. Loneliness, when seen in the right light, can become a valuable teacher, a chance to rediscover oneself and develop a sense of inner wholeness that does not rely on others.

The first step in this journey is learning to be comfortable with being alone. This doesn't mean isolation, but learning to enjoy your own company, cultivating your interests, passions, and personal growth. When we fill our time and space with things that nourish us, loneliness stops being a threat and becomes a source of strength.

Another key step is developing a healthy relationship with oneself, based on self-compassion and acceptance. Often, those who fear loneliness do so because they cannot bear to be alone with their thoughts, fears, and insecurities. But when we start to treat ourselves with love and kindness, solitude is no longer a terrifying void but a moment of intimacy with our deepest self.

- **Exercise for Positive Solitude**: Dedicate time each week to doing something you enjoy by yourself. Choose activities that excite you and allow you to connect with yourself. This will help you see solitude as an opportunity for growth rather than a condition to fear.

Conclusion: Solitude as a Tool for Autonomy

The fear of loneliness is one of the most powerful forces behind emotional dependence, but it is not a life sentence. It is a fear that can be transformed, a challenge that invites us to explore the depths of ourselves, to recognize that our worth and happiness do not depend solely on others.

When we learn to face loneliness without fear, when we accept being with ourselves and find in ourselves the source of our well-being, we can finally free ourselves from the chains of emotional dependence. Relationships no longer become a necessity to fill a void but a conscious choice, a space for

mutual growth, where love is free, mature, and no longer
governed by the fear of being alone.

The Inner Void: Seeking in Others What is Missing in Oneself

There is a profound emptiness that resides in the hearts of
many, an inner void that is often difficult to recognize and even
harder to confront. This void is not simply loneliness, nor is it
just melancholy. It is an unfathomable space, a silent crack in
our soul that compels us, sometimes without realizing it, to
desperately seek in others what we cannot find in ourselves. It
is a lack that echoes within, a sense of incompleteness that
drives many of our relationships, turning love and the desire
for closeness into emotional dependence.

Those who live with an inner void often seek in others a refuge,
a safe harbor where they can feel complete, shielded from the
turmoil of this absence they are unable to fill. The other person
becomes a kind of distorted mirror, reflecting back all the
things they feel they lack: love, security, worth. Yet, this mirror
never truly reflects our essence; instead, it returns only a
distorted image of ourselves, magnifying our deficiencies and
turning every relationship into a desperate attempt to find
externally what is missing inside.

The Inner Void: The Silent Shadow of the Soul

The inner void can arise from various experiences: the absence
of love in childhood, rejection, abandonment, or simply never
having had the opportunity to truly know and accept oneself. It
is an emotional space left empty by everything we did not
receive or by everything we somehow feel unworthy of.

This void creates a lack of identity, an inability to define oneself
without another person. Self-esteem crumbles, and one
perceives themselves as incomplete, inadequate, never
enough. It is as if a fundamental part of oneself is missing, and
we are constantly searching for something or someone to fill
that void, to provide the sense of completeness that we cannot
find alone.

In this context, relationships become a sort of emotional panacea: the other person is seen as the solution to the void, the only possible source of love, validation, and security. But this perception is deeply misleading, because the inner void cannot be filled by someone else. On the contrary, attempting to fill it through a relationship only deepens it, creating dynamics of emotional dependence where the other person becomes a necessity rather than a choice.

Projection: Idealizing the Other to Fill One's Own Gaps

Those who live with an inner void tend to idealize their partner, projecting onto them all the qualities they feel they lack. The partner is seen as perfect, as the answer to all their insecurities and fears. But this idealization is merely an illusion, a flight from reality. No person can truly meet all of our expectations or fill such a deep void. When the other inevitably fails to maintain this idealized image, the result is devastating disappointment.

Projection creates a dynamic where the partner becomes the emotional savior, someone on whom our sense of security and worth entirely depends. Every word, every gesture of the partner takes on disproportionate meaning: a signal of approval brings joy and relief, while an unspoken word, a missed attention, or a sign of emotional distance triggers fear, jealousy, and insecurity. In this way, the relationship becomes a constant emotional rollercoaster, where love is no longer experienced as a free and reciprocal bond but as a continuous attempt to fill an insatiable need.

Instead of being a life partner with whom to grow, the other person becomes a kind of lifeline, someone on whom our very ability to feel worthy depends. But this type of dynamic is fragile because it is based on a lie: the idea that the inner void can be filled from the outside when, in fact, it can only be filled by ourselves.

Emotional Dependence: Seeking Salvation in the Other

The inner void, if left unaddressed, creates the perfect conditions for emotional dependence. A dependent person does not love the other for who they are but for what they represent: a solution to their own sense of incompleteness. They cling to the partner in the hope that the relationship will provide a kind of emotional salvation, as if love could magically resolve all the insecurities and fears that reside within.

In this dynamic, the other person becomes the center of the emotional universe. The relationship is no longer an encounter between two complete individuals but a fusion in which one depends on the other to feel valid. This creates an unbalanced relationship, where one (or both) partners sacrifice their own desires and needs just to maintain the closeness of the other.

Emotional dependence leads to a loss of self, a gradual erasure of one's own identity. The dependent person stops listening to their own needs and desires, constantly adapting to the other's requirements in the hope of preserving the bond. But in this self-sacrifice, the inner void never gets filled; instead, it deepens, creating a cycle of dissatisfaction and suffering that makes it impossible to experience true, free love.

The Inner Void and the Fear of Abandonment

Another key aspect of the inner void is the constant fear of abandonment. Those who live with a sense of incompleteness tend to perceive every sign of distance or disinterest as a threat, as confirmation that the other is about to leave. Solitude is seen as unbearable because it means confronting the void they have been trying to avoid. As a result, every gesture, every word, every silence of the partner is interpreted through the lens of fear: "Do they still love me?" "Are they about to leave me?" "Am I not enough for them?"

This fear drives obsessive behaviors, such as seeking constant reassurance, controlling the partner, or doing anything to avoid conflict in the hope of keeping the relationship intact. But in this attempt to hold onto the other, freedom, authenticity, and reciprocity—the foundations of a healthy relationship—are lost.

The fear of abandonment, fueled by the inner void, creates a dynamic where the partner is always seen as unstable, as something that could be lost at any moment. This perpetual anxiety suffocates the relationship, turning love into a kind of emotional warfare to keep the other close at any cost. But true love cannot flourish when it is trapped in fear.

Filling the Void: The Path to Authenticity and True Love

To break the cycle of the inner void and emotional dependence, one must look within and confront the lack they have been avoiding for so long. This process requires courage and a deep willingness for self-exploration, as it means facing one's insecurities, fears, and emotional wounds. The inner void cannot be filled by someone else, but only by oneself, through an act of acceptance and self-love.

The first step is to learn to recognize one's intrinsic value, independent of relationships. Instead of seeking validation from others, we must develop a solid self-esteem that allows us to feel complete and worthy, even when we are alone. This does not mean living without relationships, but rather living relationships where love is a conscious choice, not an emotional survival mechanism.

- **Inner Reconnection Exercise**: Take time each day to be alone with your thoughts. Meditate, journal, or simply observe what arises from your inner world. Learn to get to know the parts of yourself that you have avoided and begin to accept them with love and compassion.

Conclusion: Love as an Encounter Between Complete Souls

The inner void is a condition that many experience, but it is not a life sentence. It is an invitation to look within, to discover who we truly are, and to find within ourselves the qualities we have so desperately sought in others. When we learn to fill our own void with authenticity and self-acceptance, relationships stop being an escape from loneliness and become a space for mutual growth, where love is free to flourish without the chains of dependence.

True love does not arise from need but from the conscious choice to share one's life with another human being while remaining true to oneself. When we learn to live in harmony with our inner selves, we can finally experience authentic relationships, where the other person is no longer seen as a solution to our deficiencies but as a companion on the journey through life's beauty.

Learning to Be Alone: Solitude as an Opportunity for Growth

Solitude, often perceived as a dark shadow following us in silence, is one of the most feared emotions. It is associated with abandonment, emptiness, and a sense of isolation, which seems to suggest the absence of connection and human warmth. Yet, behind this fear of solitude lies a deeper truth: solitude is not just a place of desolation but also a sacred space, a precious opportunity to rediscover oneself, to heal, and to grow. Learning to be alone is an art, one of the highest forms of courage and emotional maturity, because it means being able to inhabit one's inner space without fear, discovering that, in the silence and quiet, there is a vast world of discoveries.

In modern culture, which celebrates hyperconnection and constant interaction, solitude is often seen as a failure, a lack of affection, love, or belonging. But in reality, solitude is essential for our well-being, a necessary step on the path to authenticity. Only through solitude can we learn to explore the depths of our being, to engage in dialogue with ourselves, and to uncover that hidden part of ourselves that often remains in the shadows of social dynamics. Solitude, when embraced with wisdom, becomes a silent companion, guiding us toward a deeper understanding of our identity and our place in the world.

Solitude as a Meeting with Oneself

Being alone means confronting oneself without filters, without distractions, without the comfort of another's presence, which sometimes diverts us from our deepest emotions. When we are alone, there is no one to lean on, no distraction to rely on, and this can initially be frightening. It is like standing before a mirror that reflects every part of us, even those we would rather ignore: our fears, insecurities, and vulnerabilities.

But it is precisely in this meeting, in the intimate dialogue with the self, that solitude reveals its transformative power. In silence, hidden truths, unexpressed desires, and wounds that need healing emerge. It is a space where we can finally listen to ourselves without external interference, without seeking someone else's approval or judgment. It is a space of total authenticity where we can no longer pretend to be anything other than who we truly are.

Solitude invites us to reclaim our identity, to stop seeking validation from others and instead find within ourselves that spark of light that makes us unique. In this space, we can cultivate a deeper relationship with ourselves, learning to respect our needs, recognize our limits, and develop a form of self-compassion that allows us to embrace our imperfections without judgment.

Solitude as a Source of Creativity and Intuition

Solitude is not only an opportunity for introspection but also a source of creativity. When we are alone, free from the constant influence of social expectations or others' opinions, our creative spirit has room to emerge more freely and authentically. In solitude, we can explore new ideas, imagine possibilities we had not considered, and give voice to the part of us that is often stifled by the noise of the outside world.

Many great thinkers, artists, and writers have found in solitude an inexhaustible source of inspiration. In silence, a void is created in which intuitions can flourish, where the mind, liberated from distractions, can wander and discover new horizons. In this sense, solitude is fertile ground for creativity, a place where we can experiment without fear of judgment or misunderstanding.

When we are alone, we can give shape to our dreams and visions without the need to conform to what others expect from us. It is an act of inner freedom where we can experiment, fail, and grow without the pressure of always needing to be perfect or accommodating. Solitude thus becomes a space for authentic expression, where we can nurture our art, imagination, and ability to see the world in new ways.

Solitude as a Teacher of Emotional Freedom

Learning to be alone is also a fundamental step toward emotional independence. Often, in relationships, we tend to seek security and comfort in others, entrusting them with the responsibility for our happiness. But this emotional dependence, while understandable, can become a trap. When we rely entirely on another person to feel complete, we lose touch with ourselves and become vulnerable to the fear of abandonment and loneliness.

Solitude teaches us that we can find strength and comfort within ourselves, that we do not need someone else to feel worthy or complete. It teaches us that true emotional freedom comes from recognizing that we are already whole, that our happiness does not depend on external circumstances but on how we relate to ourselves. It is an act of self-affirmation, where we learn to take care of our emotional well-being without constantly depending on the presence or approval of others.

When we learn to be alone, we free ourselves from the obsessive need to fill every empty space with someone else's presence. We become capable of being in our own company, of accepting silence, and of transforming it into a resource rather than a source of fear. This emotional freedom allows us to live relationships more balanced, without the constant fear of losing the other or being abandoned.

The Inner Journey: Discovering Fullness in Solitude

Solitude is an inner journey, a path that leads us to a deeper connection with our essence. On this journey, we learn to see solitude not as a condition of deprivation but as a space of inner fullness. When we allow ourselves to inhabit our solitude, we discover that we are never truly alone because within us there is a rich and complex world, full of emotions, thoughts, dreams, and intuitions waiting to be discovered.

In this sense, solitude becomes a rite of passage, a crucial step in our personal evolution. It is an opportunity to reconnect with the part of ourselves that we too often neglect and to find in our deepest self a source of stability and strength. Solitude teaches us to recognize our intrinsic worth, beyond relationships, external validation, or circumstances.

In this quiet space, we learn to celebrate our uniqueness, to cultivate self-love, and to find meaning and fulfillment in our own presence. Solitude thus becomes a source of empowerment, a condition where we realize that we are the sole architects of our destiny and that our happiness depends primarily on our ability to be at peace with who we are.

Conclusion: Solitude as a Tool for Growth

Learning to be alone is an act of great courage, a gesture of self-love that allows us to grow and evolve. In solitude, we discover that we are not incomplete without others, but that our fullness comes from within. It is a lesson that teaches us to live relationships with greater authenticity and freedom because we no longer seek in others what we can only find in ourselves.

Solitude, therefore, is not a void to be filled but a space of opportunity, a fertile ground where we can cultivate our creativity, intuition, and spirit. It is a journey toward self-discovery, a path that leads us to greater awareness and authenticity. And when we learn to be alone, we discover that silence is never truly silent but full of voices, dreams, and possibilities waiting to be heard.

Filling the Emotional Void with Self-Compassion and Self-Esteem

There is a secret place hidden within the folds of the soul where the emotional void often takes shape. It's a space that feels devoid of warmth, where the absence of love, security, and self-esteem is felt like an open wound. This void may not always be visible from the outside, but within, it manifests as a constant feeling of incompleteness, as if something essential is missing to truly feel at home, at peace with oneself. If not addressed, this void pushes us to seek external validation, relationships to complete us, and attention to alleviate the sense of lack.

But what we seek externally is never the real answer. The emotional void cannot be filled by other people or external circumstances. The path to filling that void begins within, through the practice of self-compassion and the cultivation of self-esteem. These two tools not only help us heal, but they also transform that void into a source of inner strength, a place where self-love blooms and finally frees us from the need to seek in others what we can only find within ourselves.

The Emotional Void: A Gap to Be Filled with Love

The emotional void often manifests as a sense of inadequacy, a deeply rooted belief that we are not enough: not loved enough, not worthy enough, not strong enough. This void can stem from childhood, from missed relationships, unsaid words, or traumas that taught us to believe we lack value. It drives us to live in a state of constant search, as if only the approval of others could fill that deep absence.

Yet, the more we try to fill the void with love and approval from others, the more it seems to widen. This happens because we are seeking the solution in the wrong place. The emotional void is not a lack of external validation but a lack of self-love. The first true answer is to learn to fill that void from within, with a love that does not depend on circumstances but arises from the recognition of our intrinsic worth.

Self-Compassion: The Art of Loving Oneself in Our Wounds

The first step to filling the emotional void is the practice of self-compassion. Often, we are our harshest critics: we judge ourselves for our mistakes, punish ourselves for our weaknesses, and convince ourselves that we are never enough for our own expectations or those of others. This relentless judgment only deepens the void, making us feel constantly inadequate and lacking.

Self-compassion, on the other hand, is the ability to greet ourselves with kindness, to treat ourselves with the same understanding we would offer a dear friend. It means recognizing that our wounds, fears, and failures are part of the human experience and deserve love, not condemnation. When we grant ourselves compassion, we begin to heal that void with the awareness that, even in our imperfections, we are worthy of love and respect.

• **Self-Compassion Exercise**: Each time you notice yourself being overly critical, stop and ask yourself, "How would I treat a friend in my same situation?" Try speaking to yourself with the same words of comfort and support you would offer another person. This simple act of kindness towards yourself can begin to fill that void with a sense of warmth and acceptance.

Self-compassion is a balm for the wounded heart because it allows us to slow down and stop fighting against ourselves. It teaches us that we don't have to be perfect to be loved and that we can embrace our vulnerabilities without hiding them. In this space of acceptance, the void begins to fill with sweetness, peace, and a love that does not require conditions.

Self-Esteem: Building a Pillar of Trust in Oneself

Alongside self-compassion, self-esteem is the other essential pillar for filling the emotional void. While self-compassion teaches us to love ourselves in our weaknesses, self-esteem teaches us to believe in our worth and to cultivate deep trust in our abilities. Self-esteem does not stem from arrogance or the need to prove something to others, but from the awareness that, regardless of external circumstances, we are worthy of respect and love.

Many people who suffer from an emotional void struggle with deep insecurity, leading them to constantly doubt their qualities and seek validation from others. But self-esteem is built not through external approval but through a healthy relationship with oneself. This means learning to recognize one's strengths, celebrating successes, and accepting imperfections as part of the growth process.

• **Self-Esteem Exercise**: Every day, take time to acknowledge at least three positive things about yourself. They can be small achievements, personal qualities, or simple acts of kindness you've shown towards yourself or others. Write them down and reread them, reminding yourself that your worth is not determined by external judgments but by your ability to recognize it.

Self-esteem allows us to develop a solid foundation upon which to build our identity. When we trust ourselves, we no longer need to constantly seek others' approval to feel valid. We feel rooted in our worth, enabling us to face life with greater confidence and independence. The emotional void begins to fade, replaced by a stable, lasting presence that accompanies us even in difficult times.

Recognizing Your Intrinsic Worth

One of the most important aspects of filling the emotional void is learning to recognize your intrinsic worth, regardless of circumstances. Often, people who suffer from an emotional void feel incomplete because they measure their worth based on external factors: career success, others' approval, romantic relationships. But these are fragile confirmations that can change and disappear.

Our worth, however, is something unchanging, not dependent on our successes or failures. It is the simple fact of existing, of being unique and irreplaceable, that makes us worthy of love. When we begin to recognize this worth, the emotional void transforms into an inner fullness, an awareness that we are already complete, already enough, just as we are.

• **Value Recognition Exercise**: Take a few minutes each day to meditate or reflect on the concept of worth. Repeat to yourself, "I am worthy of love and respect, regardless of what I do or achieve." Make this affirmation a central part of your inner dialogue.

Transforming the Void into a Creative Space

The emotional void is not just an absence but can become a creative space from which transformation is born. When we stop fearing the void and begin to see it as an opportunity to fill it with love and self-esteem, a new horizon of possibilities opens up. Instead of desperately trying to fill that void with external elements, we can fill it with nourishment for the soul, through the exploration of who we are, our dreams, and our passions.

The void can become fertile ground where new meanings, new visions, and new ways of being can grow. When we fill it with self-compassion and self-esteem, we realize that the void was not a lack but an invitation to rediscover ourselves, to understand who we really are without the masks and expectations of others.

Conclusion: Filling the Void with Inner Light

Filling the emotional void with self-compassion and self-esteem is an act of inner rebirth. It is a journey that requires patience, kindness, and commitment but ultimately leads us to a fundamental truth: we are already complete, already worthy, already enough. We do not need to seek outside what we can find within.

When we learn to love ourselves in our fragility, to recognize our worth without conditions, the void naturally fills, not with external validation but with the light of our own presence. At that moment, we realize that the truest love is the love we can give ourselves, for only from there can we truly love and live with authenticity and fullness.

The Process of Awareness

The First Step Towards Healing: Recognizing the Problem

Healing is a journey that begins with an act of inner courage: recognizing the problem. This is a crucial moment, often filled with pain and resistance, because admitting that something is wrong requires us to look within with new eyes, stripped of the illusions we've built to protect ourselves. It's like breaking through the shell of an armor we've worn for so long to shield ourselves from the world and, at times, from ourselves. But that shell, now too tight, suffocates us, trapping us in a cycle of suffering that we can no longer ignore. Only then, in a moment of clear awareness, do we understand that healing cannot occur without first acknowledging the problem.

Recognizing a problem doesn't simply mean noticing or admitting its existence. It is an act of radical self-honesty, requiring us to confront the darkest and most painful parts of ourselves. It means stopping the cycle of running away, hiding, or minimizing what hurts us, and instead choosing to face reality, with all its weight. This step, which may feel fragile and uncertain, is actually the strongest foundation upon which to build the path to healing.

The Pain of Recognition: Breaking the Illusion

Recognizing a problem—whether emotional, relational, or psychological—means breaking the illusion we've built around it. For a long time, we may have tried to ignore the signs, rationalize our behavior, or convince ourselves that everything was fine, even as we felt a growing fracture in our inner balance.

These illusions often stem from fear of change or the pain of confronting the truth the problem hides. We prefer to maintain the appearance of normalcy, accepting a constant discomfort rather than facing the reality that, once revealed, might force us to transform our lives. Yet ignoring the problem doesn't make it disappear—it amplifies it, leaving it to operate in the shadows until it overwhelms us with a force we can no longer contain.

Recognizing the problem means giving voice to the pain we've ignored or repressed. It's like opening a door to an inner landscape filled with wounds, insecurities, fears, and anger that we've tried to hide. Initially, this act of recognition may seem devastating, almost as if we're admitting defeat. But in reality, this is where healing begins: only when we stop fighting against what hurts us can we begin to transform it.

The Strength of Confrontation: Facing the Problem Head-On

Facing the problem directly is an act of both strength and vulnerability. It's a moment when we stop and ask ourselves: "What is really happening inside me?" This kind of confrontation requires deep awareness, a gaze that goes beyond the surface and invites us to explore the roots of our distress.

This may mean acknowledging emotional dependency, toxic behavioral patterns, an unhealed wound, or a pain we've avoided. It's a moment where we allow ourselves to be fragile, to admit that we are not invincible, that we need help, or that we've made choices that have led us away from our true well-being.

• **Awareness Exercise**: Whenever you feel emotional discomfort, stop and ask yourself, "Where is this feeling coming from? What is it telling me?" Take the time to listen to the answers without judgment or rushing to fix them. This will help you connect with the root of the problem, opening the path to healing.

Recognizing the problem is not a sign of weakness but of maturity. It means understanding that every suffering has a source, and unless we face it, it will continue to influence our lives. It's like confronting a knot that, however difficult, must be untangled for us to move forward.

Accepting the Truth: The Weight and Freedom of Awareness

One of the hardest parts of recognizing a problem is accepting the truth it brings. Often, the pain of this awareness can feel unbearable. We may discover that the problem runs deeper than we thought, extending not only to the present but to old wounds, behavioral patterns, or limiting beliefs we've held for years.

Accepting this truth can feel like an initial defeat, as if admitting the problem also means accepting that we are fallible, vulnerable, or have made wrong choices. Yet, this is one of the highest forms of inner freedom. It is the moment when we free ourselves from the burden of always having to be strong, always maintaining a façade of perfection, and allow ourselves to be human.

Accepting the problem also means accepting that we don't need all the answers right away and that the path to healing is a process of steps, setbacks, and progress. Healing is not an instantaneous event but a journey built day by day with patience and dedication. And the recognition of the problem is the first step on this path.

• **Acceptance Exercise**: Take a moment to reflect on a difficulty you are facing. Instead of trying to change it immediately, sit with it. Accept it for what it is without trying to fix or deny it. Allow yourself to feel the emotions it brings, remembering that acceptance is not surrender but recognizing what is real.

The Power of Transformation: Recognizing to Heal

Recognizing a problem is the act that opens the door to transformation. When we finally see what hurts us, we can begin to work towards healing that wound. It's not just about admitting discomfort but embracing it with the intention to transform it. It's like looking at a devastated land and deciding to cultivate it with care, planting seeds of awareness, compassion, and love.

Healing is not a linear process. There will be moments of regression, times when the pain seems to prevail, but each time we recognize the problem, we take a step towards liberation. It's like a scar that, over time, stops hurting and becomes a symbol of our strength and journey towards healing.

Recognizing the problem doesn't mean defeating it immediately, but it does mean starting to care for it. It means making space for emotions, fears, and welcoming them as parts of us that need to be seen, understood, and healed. It's the first act of self-love, a gesture of self-compassion that says: "I see myself, I hear myself, and I am ready to heal."

Conclusion: The Courage to Look Within

Recognizing the problem is the first step towards healing, but it's also the most important. It is an act of courage that requires us to look within without fear, to confront our shadows, and to accept that, no matter how painful, only through this awareness can we truly heal. It is the moment when we stop running and start walking towards liberation.

Healing means transforming pain into wisdom, wounds into strength, and recognizing the problem is the key that opens the door to this transformation. When we choose to clearly see what hurts us, we also choose to give ourselves the opportunity to heal, grow, and live with greater authenticity and inner peace.

The Importance of Awareness of One's Inner Dynamics

There is a hidden world within each of us—a complex emotional landscape made of thoughts, sensations, and desires that flow beneath the surface, often beyond our daily consciousness. This inner world is an intricate weave of memories, emotions, and impulses that guide us, like an underground river, influencing our decisions, shaping our relationships, and coloring how we perceive the world around us. Yet, many of our actions, reactions, and choices are governed by inner dynamics of which we are not fully aware. This leads us to live in a kind of disconnection from ourselves, as if part of our existence were hidden behind a thin veil—unseen, but powerful.

Becoming aware of one's inner dynamics means looking beyond the surface, exploring the deeper layers of our being to understand what moves our emotions, fuels our fears, and drives certain behaviors. It's an act of discovery, reflection, and above all, truth. When we are aware of our inner dynamics, we are no longer victims of our automatic responses; we become active participants in our lives, capable of making authentic choices aligned with our true selves.

The Exploration of Self: A Necessary Journey

Awareness of one's inner dynamics is a journey of self-exploration that requires attention, patience, and the courage to face what we often prefer to ignore. Inner dynamics can be seen as underground currents that influence our behavior unconsciously: unexpressed emotions, unrecognized needs, beliefs we've inherited or developed over time.

These hidden mechanisms operate like repetitive patterns, leading us to react in ways we don't fully understand. Perhaps we get angry without knowing the true reason, feel insecure in situations that don't justify it, or repeatedly choose relationships or circumstances that recreate old patterns of suffering. Without awareness, these cycles repeat endlessly, dragging us into a loop of actions and reactions that deeply affect our lives.

However, when we start to observe and understand these dynamics, we can begin to break those cycles. Awareness allows us to recognize the patterns we've internalized and consciously choose how to act, rather than reacting automatically. It's like turning on a light in a dark room: only when we can clearly see what's there can we start to organize, transform what no longer serves us, and create space for a more authentic and free life.

The Connection Between Mind and Heart: Dialogue with Your Emotions

One of the most important aspects of being aware of your inner dynamics is the ability to connect with your emotions. Emotions are the language of the soul, precious messengers that show us what is happening within. Yet, we often ignore or suppress them because they seem too intense, uncomfortable, or at odds with the image we want to project to the world.

When we are not aware of our emotions, they accumulate beneath the surface, influencing our decisions in ways we do not understand. Unexpressed resentment, an unaddressed fear, or an unresolved pain manifests in automatic behaviors, anxiety, stress, or dysfunctional relationships. Emotions, when ignored, become like shadows following us everywhere, distorting our perception of the world.

Awareness of inner dynamics means accepting and listening to emotions, allowing them to emerge and reveal their messages. Each emotion has a story to tell: fear speaks of perceived threats, anger signals violated boundaries, sadness reveals what has been lost. Only by entering into dialogue with these emotions can we transform them from destructive forces into tools for growth and self-understanding.

- **Emotional Awareness Exercise**: Whenever you feel a strong emotion, pause for a moment and ask yourself, "What is this emotion trying to tell me?" Notice the sensations in your body and allow the emotion to express itself without judgment. This practice will help you develop a deeper understanding of your inner dynamics.

Limiting Beliefs: The Invisible Cage

Our inner dynamics are deeply shaped by limiting beliefs we have developed throughout life. These beliefs act like a lens through which we view the world—a lens that can distort our perception of reality. Often, we are not even aware of these beliefs because we have internalized them for so long that we regard them as absolute truths.

Beliefs such as "I'm not enough," "I don't deserve love," or "I have to be perfect to be accepted" can influence every aspect of our lives, from how we relate to others to our sense of self-worth. These beliefs form an invisible cage that limits our possibilities, keeping us trapped in negative thought patterns.

Becoming aware of our limiting beliefs is a crucial step toward freeing ourselves from them. Only when we recognize that these beliefs are the result of past experiences, family conditioning, or cultural influences can we begin to question and replace them with more positive and constructive thoughts. This process allows us to expand our view of the world and open ourselves to new possibilities for growth and fulfillment.

- **Belief Exploration Exercise**: Reflect on a challenging situation in your life and ask yourself, "What belief is influencing my behavior in this situation?" Write down the answers and try to challenge those beliefs, asking if they are truly valid or if they are the result of old mental patterns.

Integrating Awareness: The Transformation of Self

Being aware of your inner dynamics doesn't just mean recognizing what drives you—it also means integrating this awareness into your daily life. Awareness becomes a tool for transformation, allowing you to live more authentically, making choices that reflect your true self rather than being driven by fears or conditioning.

When we integrate awareness of our inner dynamics, we become better equipped to manage conflict, build healthier relationships, and live with greater emotional balance. This integration allows us to act with intention, rather than react impulsively. We choose kindness over anger, understanding over judgment. It is a process that leads us to live in greater alignment with our values and purpose, enabling us to flourish as individuals and bring more harmony to our own lives and to those around us.

Awareness of inner dynamics is an ongoing journey, a process of discovery that accompanies us throughout life. It is not a fixed destination, but a practice that invites us to stay attuned to ourselves, to accept our complexities, and to transform what limits us into a source of wisdom and growth.

Conclusion: Awareness as a Path to Freedom

Awareness of your inner dynamics is a key to liberation. When we stop being driven by our automatic responses and become aware of what is happening within, we can finally take control of our lives. Instead of being swept away by emotional currents or limiting beliefs, we can choose to navigate with intention and clarity, transforming our inner experiences into tools for evolution.

Being aware of our inner dynamics means living with integrity, in harmony with our true essence. It means learning to look within with new eyes, to explore our depths with curiosity and without fear. And in this journey toward greater awareness, we discover that within us lies a vast universe of possibilities, ready to be explored and transformed into a richer, more authentic, and freer life.

How Mindfulness Can Help Understand and Address Emotional Dependency

Emotional dependency is an invisible bond that ties us to another person, not by choice, but by need. It is an emotional prison where love is intertwined with fear—the fear of losing the other person, of being abandoned, of not being enough. In emotional dependency, the partner becomes the center of our emotional universe, a source of value and security that we believe we cannot find within ourselves. This leads to unbalanced, suffocating relationships where our identity dissolves in the attempt to keep the other person close. However, there is a way out of this prison—a path to healing that lies in the practice of mindfulness.

Mindfulness, or full awareness, is the ability to be present in the moment, to observe without judgment what happens both inside and outside of us. It is a practice of conscious attention that allows us to reconnect with ourselves, with our emotions, thoughts, and desires, without being overwhelmed by them. Through mindfulness, we can begin to explore the roots of emotional dependency, recognize the automatic mechanisms that drive us to seek in others what we lack, and develop emotional autonomy.

Mindfulness as a Tool for Self-Awareness

One of the central aspects of mindfulness is the ability to observe without judgment. This simple act of observation allows us to become witnesses to our internal experience without fully identifying with it. When we are trapped in emotional dependency, emotions like fear, jealousy, or the need for reassurance can become so intense that we feel there is no escape. In these moments, we often react impulsively: we seek reassurance, cling to the other person, or withdraw into ourselves. However, these reactions only reinforce the dynamics of dependency.

Mindfulness invites us to pause and observe what is happening inside us before reacting. Through practice, we begin to notice how emotional dependency is fueled by recurring thoughts and limiting beliefs: "I am not enough," "I need him/her to be happy," "I cannot live without the other." These thoughts trap us in a cycle of insecurity and need, making it impossible to live love authentically and freely.

Mindfulness offers us the space to recognize these thought patterns, to see them clearly, and to understand that they are not absolute truths but simply products of our mind. When we become aware of these automatic responses, we can start to detach from them, choosing not to react immediately to our impulses but to observe and understand what is truly happening within us.

• **Mindfulness Exercise**: When you feel overwhelmed by fear or anxiety in a relationship, stop for a moment and take three deep breaths. Observe the thoughts that arise and acknowledge the emotions you are feeling. Do not try to change or push them away; simply note them, as if you were watching clouds pass in the sky. This simple act of presence will help defuse automatic reactions and cultivate greater self-understanding.

The Power of the Breath: Returning to Center

In emotional dependency, we often feel as though we are out of control, as if our emotions completely dominate our lives. Every gesture, every word or silence from the partner can trigger waves of insecurity, jealousy, or fear. It is as if our inner balance is constantly at the mercy of external events, making us slaves to our emotions.

Mindfulness teaches us that the breath is an anchor, a point of return that allows us to re-center and reconnect with ourselves. When we are gripped by anxiety or fear, our breath tends to become rapid and shallow, feeding the feeling of stress. Through mindfulness, we can learn to breathe consciously, using the breath as a way to calm the mind and establish a sense of presence and stability.

Learning to return to the breath during moments of crisis helps us avoid being overwhelmed by emotions. Instead of reacting impulsively to the fear of abandonment or feelings of emptiness, we can take a few deep breaths and return to ourselves. This simple gesture helps us maintain our emotional autonomy, reminding us that we can face our emotions without being consumed by them, and that our happiness does not entirely depend on the other person.

• **Mindful Breathing Exercise**: When you feel the need for reassurance or when emotions become too intense, close your eyes and focus your attention on your breath. Breathe deeply, counting to four as you inhale, then exhale slowly, counting to four. Repeat this cycle for five breaths. This exercise will help calm the nervous system and bring you back to the present moment.

Cultivating Self-Acceptance: Self-Love Through Mindfulness

Emotional dependency often stems from a deep lack of self-esteem. When we do not feel enough, we constantly seek validation from others. We become dependent on their attention and affection because we believe that only through them can we feel complete. But this need creates a vicious cycle: the more we seek external validation, the emptier and more insecure we feel inside.

Mindfulness invites us to cultivate self-acceptance, to learn to treat ourselves with the same kindness and compassion we offer others. Through mindfulness, we can develop a closer relationship with ourselves, learning to see our imperfections and vulnerabilities and embracing them without judgment.

Being aware of ourselves allows us to recognize our intrinsic value, beyond what others think of us. Through mindfulness, we can begin to build a solid sense of self-esteem that no longer depends on external validation but on our ability to be present for ourselves, accepting who we are with all our strengths and weaknesses.

• **Self-Compassion Exercise**: Every day, take a few minutes to practice gratitude toward yourself. Close your eyes and focus on your heart. Mentally repeat: "I see myself, I accept myself, I love myself as I am." Feel these words take root within you, like a seed growing and blossoming. This exercise will help you develop a sense of love and acceptance for yourself, independent of external relationships.

Creating Space for Emotional Freedom

One of the most profound lessons mindfulness teaches us is that we can create space between ourselves and our emotions. Emotions are not permanent; they are like waves that rise and fall. When we are trapped in emotional dependency, emotions seem overwhelming, as if there is no escape. But mindfulness shows us that we can observe emotions without fully identifying with them.

Through awareness, we learn that love does not need to be based on need but on conscious choice. We can choose to love another person not out of fear or lack but because we freely choose to share our lives with them. Mindfulness allows us to see love not as a chain but as an act of freedom—a gesture born from our inner fullness, not from the fear of emptiness.

Conclusion: Mindfulness as a Path to Healing from Emotional Dependency

Mindfulness is not just a meditative practice but a way of living that helps us understand and transform the dynamics of emotional dependency. It offers us the tools to observe our thought patterns clearly, to embrace emotions without being overwhelmed by them, and to rediscover within ourselves the source of our value and happiness.

Through mindfulness, we can learn to live relationships more balanced, freeing ourselves from the constant need for reassurance and developing deep emotional autonomy. Healing from emotional dependency begins with recognizing that we are already whole, that self-love is the key to living love with others authentically and freely. In this space of awareness, love becomes a choice, not a necessity, and our lives open to new possibilities for growth and transformation.

Writing a Journal to Track Thoughts and Emotions

A journal is a window to the soul, a safe space where thoughts, often hidden in the folds of our inner world, finally find room to emerge. It is a silent companion, always ready to welcome our emotions without judgment, a blank page that fills with our words, giving voice to what we may not always dare to express aloud. In a fast-paced world dominated by superficiality, journaling is an intimate act with oneself, a moment when inner chaos can be organized, allowing us to observe with greater clarity what is happening within us.

Tracking thoughts and emotions through writing is not just an exercise in expression but a process of awareness that allows us to explore our deeper dynamics. The journal becomes a sort of map of the soul, a place where we can observe the fluctuations of our emotions, recognize recurring thoughts, and identify behavioral patterns that often escape our attention. Through writing, we can begin to decipher our inner world, understanding the roots of our suffering while celebrating our joys and discovering new possibilities for growth.

The Power of Writing: A Journey of Inner Discovery

Writing in a journal is not just a mechanical act but a true practice of self-reflection. Every word we put on paper becomes a bridge toward a deeper understanding of ourselves, a way to organize our thoughts and give shape to the emotions we often feel but cannot describe. In the act of writing, we connect with what is happening inside us: emotions find a voice, thoughts flow, and, in the clarity of the page, we discover parts of ourselves that often remain submerged in the unconscious.

When we sit down to write, we pause to observe what we are feeling at that very moment: what is troubling us? What brings us joy? What scares us? Through writing, we can examine our emotions without being overwhelmed, distilling inner chaos into a narrative that helps us better understand our emotional life. Every sentence written becomes a trail that guides us through the labyrinth of our feelings, helping us find meaning, understand the source of certain fears, or why we cling to certain thoughts.

Monitoring Thoughts: Recognizing Inner Patterns

One of the most important aspects of keeping a journal is the ability to monitor the thoughts that arise day after day. Often, we do not realize how deeply our thoughts influence our emotional state and actions. Thoughts can be subtle, almost imperceptible, but they hold enormous power in shaping our internal reality. A journal allows us to capture them on paper, making them visible so they can be examined more clearly.

Monitoring your thoughts means recognizing those recurring patterns that repeat over time. Thoughts of insecurity, such as "I'm not enough," or fear, like "I'm afraid of being abandoned," often guide our emotions and decisions. But when we write them down, when we observe them without judging, we can begin to understand that they are not absolute truths, but simply constructions of the mind.

Journaling is like having a mirror to the soul, a place where we can see our thoughts reflected more objectively. Once recognized, we can begin to question them, asking: "Does this thought serve me? Does it help me grow or keep me trapped in a cycle of suffering?" Through this practice, we learn not to be slaves to our thoughts but to consciously choose which ones to nurture and which to let go.

• **Thought Monitoring Exercise**: Each evening, take a few minutes to write down the most recurring thoughts of the day. Do not judge them or try to change them, just observe them as if you were an outside observer. Notice which thoughts bring you peace and which ones fuel anxiety or insecurity. Over time, this exercise will help you identify limiting thoughts and develop greater awareness of your inner dynamics.

Exploring Emotions: Giving Voice to the Unspoken

Emotions are the heart of our human experience, yet they often go misunderstood or repressed. Some emotions are so intense or uncomfortable that we prefer not to face them: fear, anger, sadness. But it is precisely these emotions, if unrecognized, that tend to flood our inner life, subtly and insidiously influencing our well-being. The journal then becomes a sacred space where we can give voice to these emotions, exploring them without fear.

Writing down the emotions we experience is like opening a window onto a rich and complex inner landscape. Through writing, we can begin to dialogue with our emotions, discovering that behind each one is a message, a hidden need waiting to be heard. Anger, for example, may indicate a boundary that has been violated; sadness may reveal a loss we have not yet processed; fear may suggest we are facing something unknown.

Tracking emotions in a journal allows us to welcome them without pushing them away or judging them. More than anything else, journaling teaches us that emotions, like waves, rise and then fall. They are not permanent but flows of energy that move through our body and mind. Writing about emotions helps us stay present with what we feel, without being overwhelmed by them, but learning to accept them as part of our human experience.

• **Emotion Monitoring Exercise**: Each morning or evening, take some time to write about the emotions you experienced during the day. What did you feel? Where did you feel those emotions in your body? Try to explore why these emotions arose, asking yourself what they stem from and what they are telling you. This exercise will help you develop greater emotional intelligence and better understand your reactions.

Transformation Through Writing: The Journal as a Tool for Growth

Journaling is not only an act of reflection but also a tool for transformation. Through writing, we can begin to chart a path toward healing and change. Tracking thoughts and emotions allows us to understand what patterns keep us stuck, but it also gives us the opportunity to imagine new ways of being.

The journal is a space where we can create new stories about ourselves. If we realize that certain recurring thoughts are harmful, we can begin to replace them with more positive and constructive ones. If we recognize that certain emotions dominate us, we can explore new ways of responding to them. The journal thus becomes a space for experimentation, where we can imagine new possibilities and develop greater emotional resilience.

• **Transformation Through Writing Exercise**: After monitoring your thoughts and emotions for a few days, try to identify a recurring pattern that limits you. Write a reflection on how you can transform that thought or emotion into something positive. Imagine an alternative, a new narrative of yourself. Write this new story as if you were writing the next chapter of your life.

Conclusion: The Journal as a Mirror of the Soul

Writing a journal to monitor thoughts and emotions is an act of self-love. It is a practice that invites us to be honest with ourselves, to acknowledge our vulnerabilities, and to celebrate our strengths. It is a sacred space where we can explore our inner world with curiosity, without fear, and where we can chart a path toward greater awareness and freedom.

The journal becomes a mirror of the soul, a traveling companion that helps us better understand who we are and who we can become. Through writing, we learn to know our depths, to understand our desires, and to heal our wounds. And, page after page, we discover that true transformation comes not from running away from ourselves but from embracing every part of who we are, with love and awareness.

Breaking the Cycle of Emotional Dependency

How to Establish Healthy Boundaries in Relationships

Relationships, like a garden, thrive when nurtured with care and love but can wither if neglected or allowed to grow uncontrollably. Boundaries within relationships are like invisible hedges that define this garden, protecting the sacred space of individuality and allowing the bond to grow in a healthy and harmonious way. Establishing healthy boundaries in relationships doesn't mean building walls or isolating oneself but rather defining areas of mutual respect where each person can flourish without invading or stifling the other.

Healthy boundaries are essential for ensuring that emotional needs, desires, and personal limits are recognized and respected. Without boundaries, relationships risk becoming toxic and imbalanced, where one partner may end up sacrificing their identity or well-being to maintain closeness with the other. On the contrary, with clear and healthy boundaries, relationships thrive, as both individuals know they have their own space and can express themselves without fear of judgment or rejection.

The Importance of Boundaries: Protecting the Integrity of the Self

Establishing healthy boundaries is an act of care for oneself and for the other. It is the awareness that, while being emotionally connected, each person in a relationship is an individual with their own needs, desires, and limits. Boundaries are not barriers that separate us from others but a way to preserve our identity within the relationship, allowing us to love and be loved in a balanced way.

Without clear boundaries, there is a risk of being in relationships where one partner constantly sacrifices to please the other, losing touch with their own desires and needs. This can create a dynamic of imbalance and resentment, where one person ends up feeling suffocated or exploited. In contrast, when boundaries are respected, each partner can express their needs without feeling guilty or selfish, and the other can respond with respect and understanding.

Knowing Yourself: The First Step in Setting Boundaries

The first step to establishing healthy boundaries in relationships is learning to know yourself. Often, we are unaware of our limits until we exceed them, until we feel that emotional saturation that tells us we have given too much or allowed someone to invade our inner space.

To establish healthy boundaries, we must ask ourselves: *What makes me feel comfortable? What are my essential needs? What makes me feel uneasy or suffocated?* These questions are fundamental to understanding where to draw the line between what is acceptable and what is not. Awareness of our emotional needs is the foundation of any balanced relationship. Only when we are in touch with our desires can we communicate them clearly and assertively.

• **Self-reflection exercise**: Take a moment to reflect on an important relationship in your life. What situations make you feel vulnerable or insecure? Are there times when you've felt the need to protect your space but didn't? This exercise will help you identify areas where clearer boundaries are needed.

The Art of Saying "No": Assertiveness as a Tool for Authenticity

Saying "no" is often one of the greatest challenges in relationships, especially for those who are used to pleasing others to avoid conflict or out of fear of rejection. However, knowing how to say "no" clearly and kindly is one of the most important aspects of setting healthy boundaries. A "no" said with love and respect is not a rejection of the other person but a way to affirm your own needs and protect your well-being.

Assertiveness is the ability to express your thoughts and feelings clearly, directly, and respectfully. Being assertive does not mean being aggressive or selfish but knowing how to communicate what you feel honestly and authentically without fear of how the other will react. Saying "no" when something makes you uncomfortable is an act of authenticity because it allows you to stay true to yourself and not sacrifice your needs to please the other.

• **Assertiveness exercise**: Think about a recent situation where you said "yes" to something you didn't want to do. Reflect on how you could have expressed a "no" in a kind but firm way. The next time you find yourself in a similar situation, practice this ability to express your limits clearly and respectfully.

Communicating Your Boundaries: The Importance of Transparency

Once we have identified our limits, it is essential to communicate them to the other person. Many misunderstandings in relationships arise because boundaries are not expressed clearly. When we expect the other person to guess what we need or automatically understand our limits, we create fertile ground for resentment and disappointment.

Communicating your boundaries means being transparent about your needs without expecting the other to automatically understand them. This can be difficult, especially when we fear the other person may feel hurt or rejected. But healthy boundaries are not a rejection of the other; rather, they are a way to ensure that the relationship remains respectful and authentic.

Empathetic communication is essential for establishing healthy boundaries. When we communicate our needs, it's important to do so in a way that the other person understands that our desire for space or protection is not a critique of the relationship but a way to ensure that both partners feel safe and respected.

• **Boundary communication exercise**: Think of a situation where you feel the need to set a boundary but are unsure how to communicate it. Write a message you would like to say to the other person, clearly expressing your need without accusing or blaming. This will help you find the right words and express yourself more clearly when it's time to have the conversation.

Mutual Respect: Cultivating a Healthy Relationship

Establishing healthy boundaries in relationships is not just about protecting your space but also respecting the boundaries of the other person. Every relationship is a delicate balance between autonomy and intimacy, and for a relationship to thrive, both partners must feel free to express their needs and respect the needs of the other.

When boundaries are respected, a safe space is created where both partners can grow and flourish. Mutual respect is the foundation of every healthy relationship: recognizing that the other person has different needs from ours, that they may have different timelines, desires, and spaces they require, is a sign of genuine love. Respecting boundaries doesn't mean distancing yourself from the other person but allowing them to be themselves within the relationship.

• **Mutual respect exercise**: Reflect on an important relationship in your life and ask yourself: "Do I respect the other person's boundaries? Are there situations where I could be more attentive to their needs?" This exercise will help you develop greater awareness of mutual respect within the relationship.

Conclusion: Boundaries as a Space for Freedom and Love

Establishing healthy boundaries in relationships is an act of love for both yourself and the other. It's the understanding that love doesn't require sacrifice or fusion but can only flourish when both partners are free to be authentic, respected, and protected in their personal space. Boundaries are the foundation of a balanced relationship because they allow each person to fully express their identity without fear of losing the other.

Through self-awareness, assertiveness, and empathetic communication, we can build relationships where love grows in a healthy and harmonious way, where intimacy is nurtured by respect and mutual understanding. In this safe space, we can love each other without losing ourselves, grow without stifling each other, and create deep and lasting connections based on trust, freedom, and genuine love.

Strategies for Leaving Toxic or Codependent Relationships

Relationships are like delicate threads that weave through our emotional lives, intertwining experiences, emotions, and bonds. However, not all relationships are meant to nourish our spirit. Some can become like invisible chains—unhealthy or codependent ties that trap us in dynamics of suffering, manipulation, and sacrifice. When a relationship becomes a weight dragging us down, constantly questioning our emotional and mental well-being, it's crucial to recognize the need for liberation. Leaving a toxic or codependent relationship is an act of deep courage—a journey toward freedom, self-love, and rediscovering who we truly are.

But how do we leave a relationship that, despite its destructiveness, often feels impossible to abandon? The key lies in awakening awareness, recognizing destructive dynamics, and implementing strategies to help rebuild emotional autonomy. This journey can be painful and complex, but it's a path of healing and personal redemption, where every step toward freedom is a step toward a more authentic and serene life.

1. Recognizing a Toxic or Codependent Relationship: Awakening Awareness

The first step in leaving a toxic or codependent relationship is acknowledging that the relationship itself is harmful. Often, those in toxic relationships are unaware of the severity of the situation because the dynamics of power, manipulation, or dependency are so deeply ingrained that they seem normal. Signs of a toxic relationship may include control, emotional manipulation, constant self-sacrifice for the other, a lack of respect for personal boundaries, and a pervasive feeling of anxiety or insecurity.

Codependency, on the other hand, occurs when both individuals in the relationship become emotionally dependent on one another, feeding each other's needs for validation and acceptance. In these relationships, individual identity dissolves, and emotional well-being depends entirely on the other, creating a cycle of mutual need that perpetuates itself.

To break free from these dynamics, it's essential to become aware. This means pausing and honestly examining the relationship: *How do I truly feel? What are my unmet needs? Am I sacrificing myself to maintain this relationship?* Only through this awakening can we begin to recognize that something needs to change.

• **Self-awareness exercise**: Take time to reflect on your relationship and write a list of situations where you've felt manipulated, diminished, or disrespected. Ask yourself how you really feel in the relationship and whether your needs are being met. This exercise will help you focus on the toxic or codependent dynamics that you may not have fully recognized.

2. Reclaiming Control of Your Life: Rediscovering Your Identity

One of the main characteristics of toxic or codependent relationships is the loss of identity. When we're involved in a relationship that consumes us, we often lose touch with who we really are. Our desires, dreams, and needs get smothered under the weight of the need to please the other, to maintain the relationship at all costs. To break free from a toxic relationship, it's essential to rediscover your individuality and reconnect with your true self.

Reclaiming control of your life means starting to take back your time, passions, and goals. It's an act of self-redemption that allows you to remember that your value doesn't depend on the other person but is inherent. In this process, it's important to put yourself back at the center of your life, dedicating time to personal growth and emotional and physical well-being.

• **Self-reconnection exercise**: Make a list of things you love to do but have neglected in the relationship. Dedicate time to yourself each day to cultivate these activities, which can be small daily gestures like reading, walking in nature, or pursuing a hobby. This will help you remember that your life is much more than a relationship and that you deserve to nurture your desires and dreams.

3. Setting Clear Boundaries: Protecting Your Emotional Space

One of the main reasons toxic or codependent relationships thrive is the lack of boundaries. In these relationships, personal boundaries are often violated or ignored, and the other person ends up invading your emotional, physical, or mental space. Setting clear boundaries is an act of self-protection, a way to reaffirm your dignity and worth.

Boundaries are not impenetrable walls but rather areas of mutual respect that allow us to maintain our individuality within the relationship. Setting boundaries means learning to say *no* when something isn't aligned with your needs or values and doing so kindly but firmly. Boundaries are the foundation on which a more balanced and respectful relational life can be built.

• **Boundary-setting exercise**: Reflecting on your relationship dynamics, identify a situation where you feel your boundaries have been disrespected. Write how you wish you had responded and what you could have done to protect your emotional space. Practice this response by imagining expressing your limits clearly and assertively. When a similar situation arises in the future, you will already know how to act.

4. Building a Support Network: Don't Leave Alone

Leaving a toxic or codependent relationship is a difficult and painful process, and it's essential not to go through it alone. Often, those in such relationships feel isolated, trapped in a world where the partner has taken control of their social, emotional, and even mental life. In these cases, it's crucial to rebuild a support network of friends, family, or professionals who can offer listening, understanding, and encouragement.

A support network helps maintain perspective, see the situation more clearly, and feel less alone on the journey. Those around us can act as mirrors that reflect the reality we often can't see clearly when immersed in a toxic relationship. A sincere friend or therapist can provide tools and strength to recognize dysfunctional patterns and guide us toward freedom.

• **Building a support network exercise**: Make a list of people you trust who can offer emotional support. Reach out to these people and share your situation with them, even if just for a nonjudgmental listening ear. If necessary, consider seeking the support of a therapist or counselor who can help you process your feelings and make conscious choices.

5. Letting Go: The Art of Freeing Yourself from Emotional Dependency

One of the hardest aspects of leaving a toxic or codependent relationship is letting go. Letting go isn't just about ending the relationship; it's also about facing the fears and emotional dependencies that kept you tied to the other person. Often, the fear of loneliness, failure, or emptiness prevents us from taking the step toward freedom. But letting go is an act of trust in yourself and in life.

Emotional dependency feeds on the belief that we cannot be happy or complete without the other. Letting go means reclaiming your emotional autonomy, learning to be okay on your own, and cultivating self-love that doesn't depend on external sources. This doesn't happen overnight, but it's a gradual process of healing and rebuilding self-esteem.

• **Letting go exercise**: Every day, take a few minutes to visualize yourself free from the toxic relationship. Imagine yourself walking toward a new life, lighter and full of possibilities.

Repeat mentally: *"I am whole. I am capable of loving and being loved. I lovingly free myself from what holds me back."* This exercise will help strengthen your ability to let go and build a new life.

Conclusion: The Path to Freedom and Self-Love

Leaving a toxic or codependent relationship is an act of deep courage and self-love. It's a journey that takes time, awareness, and inner strength, but it's also a path of liberation, where we learn to recognize our worth and build a life based on authenticity and balance. Through the awakening of awareness, the rebuilding of identity, the support of loved ones, and the ability to set healthy boundaries, we can regain our emotional freedom and move toward healthier, more nurturing relationships.

This healing process doesn't mean closing off your heart but instead opening it to new possibilities, to a love that is not based on fear or dependency but on conscious choice and mutual respect. In the act of letting go, we finally find our true strength: the ability to be ourselves—free and whole.

Practices for Building Emotional Autonomy: Learning to Take Care of Yourself There is an ancient wisdom that says the first true act of love is not found in gestures toward others, but in the ability to take care of oneself. In a world often dominated by expectations, complicated relationships, and constant external demands, developing emotional autonomy becomes one of the greatest and most liberating achievements we can make. Emotional autonomy is not synonymous with isolation, but a state in which our inner well-being does not depend on others, but on our ability to nurture and cultivate what we need.Learning to take care of yourself means recognizing your intrinsic value, understanding your needs, and developing a deep intimacy with yourself that can sustain you even in the most difficult moments. In this process, it's not about avoiding or rejecting relationships, but about entering them with a new awareness: the awareness that we can love and be loved without losing our center, without seeking in others the confirmation of who we are or the meaning of our existence.

1 **Cultivating Self-Awareness: The First Step Towards Emotional Autonomy**To build emotional autonomy, the first step is to learn to know yourself. This means developing a deep awareness of what we feel, how we react to situations, and what our most authentic needs are. Very often, we get lost in the hectic pace of daily life or in relational dynamics, forgetting to listen to our emotions and the signals of our body.Cultivating self-awareness is an act of presence, in which we learn to stop and listen. When we are aware of what is happening inside us, we can begin to recognize our emotional and physical needs, without waiting for someone else to fill that void. This awareness allows us to anticipate moments of discomfort, to recognize when we feel neglected or overwhelmed, and to act proactively to take care of ourselves.

- **Self-awareness exercise:** Every day, take a few minutes to stop and ask yourself: "How do I feel right now? What do I need?" Don't try to judge or change what you feel, just listen. This simple exercise in presence will help you develop a deeper connection with your emotions and recognize your needs before they become urgent or unbearable.

2 **The Practice of Self-Compassion: Treating Yourself with Kindness**Self-compassion is one of the fundamental pillars of building emotional autonomy. Very often, we are our harshest critics, scolding ourselves for every mistake, every weakness, or for not living up to expectations (our own or others'). This negative inner dialogue not only undermines our self-esteem, but makes us dependent on external validation, constantly seeking approval and affection.Learning to treat yourself with kindness means directing the same love and understanding towards yourself that you reserve for others. It's a deep act of care, which helps us see our flaws and vulnerabilities not as something to hide, but as part of our humanity. When we are capable of being compassionate toward ourselves, we can face life's difficulties without feeling overwhelmed, knowing that we have within us the ability to comfort and support ourselves.

- **Self-compassion exercise:** Whenever you feel frustrated or dissatisfied, imagine speaking to yourself as you would to a dear friend. Take time to acknowledge your fatigue or sadness and offer yourself comforting words, such as: "It's okay to feel this way. I'm doing my best, and that's enough." This simple act of kindness can make a big difference in how you deal with emotional challenges.

3 **Recognizing and Embracing Your Emotions: The Path to Healing** To build true emotional autonomy, it's essential to learn to recognize and embrace your emotions, rather than avoiding or suppressing them. Emotions are our internal guidance system: they tell us what's right and what's wrong, what nourishes us and what drains us. However, many people, out of fear of feeling pain or vulnerability, tend to stifle their emotions, seeking to fill that void with relationships or distractions. Recognizing your emotions means being honest with yourself, admitting when you are sad, angry, scared, or lonely, and giving these emotions the space to be felt. Only by embracing our emotions can we truly begin to heal our emotional wounds and build a sense of inner stability that doesn't depend on external circumstances.

- **Emotional acceptance exercise:** When you experience a strong emotion, rather than trying to push it away, stop and listen to it. Ask yourself: "What is this emotion trying to tell me? What do I need right now?" Let the emotion emerge without judging it or trying to change it. This will help you develop a healthier relationship with your emotional world, and not depend on others for comfort or validation.

4 **Building Self-Confidence: The Power of Self-Esteem** Emotional autonomy is based on self-confidence, the awareness that we have within us the resources to face difficulties and to meet our emotional needs. A lack of self-confidence makes us vulnerable to emotional dependency, because we seek in others a confirmation of our worth or our ability to handle life. Building self-confidence means recognizing your own worth, developing an esteem rooted not in external circumstances, but in your essence. Self-confidence does not arise from arrogance, but from the

awareness that we are capable of facing difficulties, of relying on ourselves, and of learning from our mistakes. Every small challenge overcome, every decision made with courage, contributes to strengthening this inner confidence, allowing us to move through the world with greater security and emotional independence.

- **Self-esteem building exercise:** Every evening, take time to reflect on three things you did well during the day, even if they are small. Acknowledge your effort, your strength, and your worth in each gesture. This will help you build a solid foundation of self-esteem, which does not depend on external approval.

5 Creating Healthy Boundaries: Protecting Your Emotional

SpaceAnother essential aspect of building emotional autonomy is learning to set healthy boundaries. Boundaries are the invisible lines that protect our emotional, physical, and mental space. Without boundaries, we risk losing ourselves in the needs of others, sacrificing our own needs to maintain peace or avoid conflict. Setting clear boundaries is an act of respect for yourself and for others.Creating healthy boundaries means knowing when to say no, knowing when it's time to take time for yourself, and communicating your needs assertively. It's not an act of selfishness, but a form of self-care that allows us to maintain our emotional integrity, even in the most intimate relationships.

- **Boundary-setting exercise:** Think of a recent situation where you felt the need to protect your emotional space but didn't. Reflect on it and imagine how you could have expressed your limits clearly and respectfully. Practice this response in your mind, so that you feel more confident the next time you need to set a boundary.

6 Caring for Yourself Physically and Emotionally: Creating Self-Care

RitualsTaking care of yourself doesn't just mean recognizing and managing your emotions, but also cultivating physical and mental well-being through self-care practices. This can include activities that nourish the body, such as a balanced diet, physical exercise, adequate rest, but also activities that nourish the spirit, such as meditation, reading, or spending time in nature. Creating personal care rituals helps us stay connected to ourselves and maintain our emotional balance.When we take care of ourselves, we send a clear message to our subconscious: "I am worthy. I deserve love, attention, and respect." This strengthens our self-esteem and allows us to enter relationships from a place of fullness, rather than from a place of lack or need.

- **Self-care exercise:** Every week, plan at least one moment of care for yourself. Whether it's a relaxing bath, a walk in nature, or simply reading a book you love, dedicate this time to yourself, without guilt. This will help you strengthen your relationship with yourself and develop greater emotional autonomy.

Conclusion: The Path to Emotional Autonomy Building emotional autonomy is a journey of rediscovery and healing, a path that leads us to become the guardians of our well-being. It's a process that requires patience, awareness, and a constant commitment to taking care of oneself, both physically and emotionally. When we learn to nurture our inner world, to recognize and respect our needs, and to treat ourselves with compassion, we become capable of living relationships more balanced, free from dependency and expectations.Emotional autonomy is not a destination, but a daily practice of self-love. It's the ability to find within ourselves the source of our security, peace, and happiness, knowing that, while we love and live with others, our center remains firm and steady, rooted in our essence.

External Support: Individual Therapy, Couples Therapy, and Support Groups On the journey toward personal growth and emotional healing, there are times when, no matter how much we work on ourselves, we realize that our pain is too deep, our wounds too ingrained, or our relational dynamics too complex to handle alone. It is during these moments that external support becomes a valuable resource, a beacon that guides us through emotional storms, offering tools, understanding, and a safety net to lean on.External support can take many forms: individual therapy, couples therapy, and support groups are powerful tools that help us explore and understand our emotional and relational dynamics, providing us with a safe space to heal and grow. These paths are not just an opportunity to resolve conflicts or traumas, but also represent a journey of self-exploration, where we can discover parts of ourselves that we may have never recognized, parts that ask to be heard, understood, and accepted.

1 **Individual Therapy: A Journey of Healing and Self-Rediscovery**Individual therapy is an intimate encounter with ourselves, guided by a professional who helps us explore our inner world with care and attention. It is a protected space where we can open the doors to our deepest feelings, confronting our fears, insecurities, traumas, and desires. Often, the emotions that dominate us or the dynamics that prevent us from living healthy and fulfilling relationships have deep roots, perhaps stemming from our childhood or past experiences that we have never fully processed.Through individual therapy, we can learn to understand the causes of certain behaviors or thought patterns that limit us, and begin to transform them. A therapist offers a safe mirror, a space for reflection free from judgment, where we can express what we feel and find new ways to respond to our emotions and the situations that trouble us.The therapeutic relationship is a special bond, built on trust and openness. Through it, we can develop greater self-awareness, learning to recognize our needs and meet them in healthier ways. Individual therapy not only helps us heal past wounds but also provides us with practical tools to face everyday challenges, cultivating an inner strength that makes us less dependent on the approval or love of others.

- **Personal reflection exercise:** If you are considering starting individual therapy, ask yourself which areas of your life you feel unable to manage alone. What emotions or behaviors seem out of control? Writing down these reflections can help clarify your thoughts and better prepare you for the therapeutic work.

2 **Couples Therapy: Rebuilding Communication and Intimacy**Couples therapy is an opportunity to rediscover and transform the emotional bond between two people. When the dynamics of a relationship become toxic or co-dependent, or when

conflicts seem insurmountable, couples therapy offers a neutral and safe space where both partners can explore their feelings and expectations. In this setting, the couple is guided to communicate more openly and respectfully, to listen to each other without prejudice, and to rebuild the foundations of a relationship based on trust and reciprocity.Couples therapy is not just for couples in crisis but can also be a preventive tool, a way to improve the quality of the relationship and address problems before they become too deeply rooted. In a couple's life, sometimes routine, misunderstandings, or unmet needs can create a distance that seems impossible to bridge. A couples therapist helps identify dysfunctional communication patterns, encouraging each partner to take responsibility for their own emotions and actions without falling into the trap of mutual blame.One of the most valuable aspects of couples therapy is the opportunity to recognize one's own boundaries and those of the other, learning to respect them without feeling threatened. It is a process that invites each partner to rediscover emotional autonomy within the relationship, allowing love to flow more freely and authentically, without the fear of losing oneself or losing the other.

- **Couples reflection exercise:** If you feel your relationship needs external support, try talking to your partner openly and honestly. Ask: "How do you really feel in our relationship? What do you think we could do together to improve our bond?" This conversation can be the first step in assessing whether couples therapy might be helpful.

3 **Support Groups: The Power of Sharing**Support groups offer a unique healing experience, based on collective sharing and mutual empathy. Being part of a support group means entering a space of listening and exchange with people who are facing situations similar to ours, who understand our difficulties without the need for long or complex explanations. There is an inherent power in sharing pain, allowing each person to feel less alone, less isolated in their journey of suffering.In support groups, the experiences of others become a source of inspiration and strength. Hearing that someone else has faced a

difficulty similar to ours and emerged stronger can give us the courage to do the same. The group becomes a support network, where everyone offers their own wisdom and life experience, and where the importance of active listening and emotional solidarity is learned.Support groups not only help process pain or relational conflicts but also provide practical tools for improving our emotional well-being. Participants, under the guidance of a facilitator or therapist, learn to manage stress, develop healthier relational skills, and recognize their own dysfunctional patterns. This process of sharing reminds us that, despite our differences, we are all united by the common desire to grow and heal.

- **Support group exploration exercise:** If you're considering joining a support group, start by researching local or online groups that address your specific issues (e.g., emotional dependency, toxic relationships, or co-dependency). Reflect on how it might be helpful to share your experience in a safe and welcoming environment, and what you hope to gain from this sharing.

4 **The Importance of External Support: An Act of Courage and Care**Seeking external support, whether through individual therapy, couples therapy, or support groups, is an act of courage and authenticity. Many people fear asking for help, afraid of being judged as weak or inadequate. But recognizing that we need support is actually one of the strongest steps we can take toward healing. It means acknowledging that we don't have to face everything alone, that there are tools and resources available to help us overcome difficulties.External support not only helps us manage emotional or relational crises but also offers us a new perspective, a broader and more compassionate view of ourselves. Through the guidance of a therapist or the exchange with a group of people sharing our path, we learn to see our difficulties not as a sign of weakness, but as opportunities for growth. This allows us to develop greater self-esteem and cultivate emotional resilience that will accompany us through all of life's challenges.

- **Opening to support exercise:** If you feel ready to seek external support, take some time to reflect on which tools might be most suitable for you: individual therapy, couples therapy, or a support group. Write down your thoughts and what you hope to gain from this journey. This will help clarify your intentions and take the first step toward greater emotional serenity.

Conclusion: A Path of Collective and Individual Growth External support, in the form of therapy or support groups, is a valuable tool for personal and relational transformation. Through the help of professionals and sharing with others, we can learn to better understand ourselves, heal our wounds, and build healthier, more fulfilling relationships. This path is not an easy road, but it is a journey of growth, authenticity, and courage, where we learn to be the protagonists of our well-being without fear of asking for help when needed.In every step toward healing, we are reminded that we are not alone. The world is full of resources, of outstretched hands ready to accompany us toward a life of greater serenity and authenticity. And when we accept this help, we open ourselves to a new phase of our journey, one where we can finally recognize our value, our strength, and our right to live a life filled with love and peace.

Part 4: Breaking Free from Emotional DependencyChapter 12

Cultivating Healthy Relationships

Building Relationships Based on Respect, Trust, and Reciprocity Relationships, like invisible threads that connect us to others, are one of the most precious and delicate aspects of our lives. Through them, we experience human connection, love, collaboration, but also challenge and growth. However, for a relationship to truly flourish, it cannot be built solely on affection or initial passion; it must rest on three fundamental pillars: respect, trust, and reciprocity. These values are not merely occasional ingredients, but rather the deep roots that sustain every lasting relationship, offering stability even through emotional storms.Building healthy relationships requires commitment, awareness, and an open heart. It is not about avoiding conflicts or seeking perfection, but about learning to nurture the bond day by day, with concrete acts of respect, with the mutual trust that is earned and renewed, and with a continuous exchange of support, love, and understanding. Relationships like this are not only a source of well-being, but also a safe haven, a space where each person can be themselves without fear, knowing they will be accepted and respected in their authenticity.

1 **Respect: The Foundation of Love and Freedom**Respect is the cornerstone of every healthy and authentic relationship. It is an act of acknowledgment, a silent declaration that says: "I see you. I recognize your worth and I respect it." Respect means accepting the other person in their entirety, with their strengths and vulnerabilities, without trying to change or mold them according to your own expectations. It is the fertile ground on which true love can grow because without respect, love turns into control, and the relationship becomes a power struggle.Respecting someone also means respecting their boundaries—physical, emotional, and mental. This not only allows the other person to feel safe but also creates a space where both people can grow without feeling suffocated. Respect is not limited to grand gestures but is most often shown in small daily actions: listening without interrupting, recognizing the other's needs without judgment, and treating them with dignity even in moments of disagreement.Respect is, ultimately, an act of mutual freedom. In a relationship based on respect, neither partner feels obligated to sacrifice their identity to maintain closeness with the other. Each is free to express themselves and be who they are, knowing the other will welcome them with kindness and openness.

- **Reflection exercise on respect:** Take time to reflect on your most important relationships. Ask yourself: "Am I respecting the other person's boundaries? Do I recognize and accept their differences without trying to change them?" Make a list of things you can do to show more respect in small, everyday actions.

2 **Trust: The Invisible Glue of Relationships**If respect is the foundation of a relationship, trust is the glue that holds it together. Trust is the deep feeling of being able to rely on the other person, of knowing that, no matter what happens, the other will not betray your vulnerability. It is

the ground on which true emotional intimacy is built because only when we trust can we lower our defenses and allow the other to see who we really are.Trust is not built in a day; it is a slow process made up of consistent and coherent actions. It arises from transparency, from the ability to be honest and communicate openly about one's feelings and thoughts. When we hide parts of ourselves or avoid facing problems, we undermine the other person's trust. On the contrary, trust is strengthened every time we choose to be authentic and to talk about even the most difficult things, knowing the other will listen with respect.But trust is not just about words; it is also demonstrated through concrete actions. It is manifested in the ability to keep promises, to be present in times of need, and to respect the implicit agreements that govern every relationship. In a relationship built on trust, there are no power games or manipulations—just a deep desire to protect and honor the connection that has been built together.

- **Trust exercise:** Reflect on how trust is manifested in your relationship. Are there areas where you could be more open or honest? Write a letter, even just for yourself, expressing how you feel about trust in your relationship and what you could do to strengthen it.

3 **Reciprocity: The Harmony of Emotional Exchange**Reciprocity is what transforms a relationship into a meeting of souls. It is the fluid and natural exchange of affection, support, understanding, and commitment between two people. In a reciprocal relationship, there is no single giver or receiver—both partners contribute equally, nurturing the bond through acts of love and generosity, without expecting anything in return but knowing the other will do the same for them.Reciprocity does not mean counting exactly what we give and receive, but rather an emotional balance in which both people feel nourished and respected. A relationship cannot last if one partner is always the one making sacrifices, or if one constantly feels neglected. Mutual generosity is what sustains the bond and makes it stable over time, allowing each person to give and receive love without feeling

drained.Reciprocity is also an act of humility. It means recognizing that, while we are strong and independent, we need others. In a healthy relationship, each partner is willing to lean on the other in times of difficulty, but also to offer support with empathy and without expecting anything in return. This exchange creates a harmonious dance in which both partners grow together, learning to balance their own needs with those of the other.

- **Reciprocity exercise:** Ask yourself if there is balance in giving and receiving in your relationship. Do you feel as supported as you support the other? Write a list of gestures of affection or support that you could offer your partner without expecting anything in return, simply for the pleasure of giving.

4 **Building Conscious Relationships: A Daily Commitment**Building relationships based on respect, trust, and reciprocity is a process that requires awareness, commitment, and time. These three pillars are not rigid rules but attitudes that are cultivated day by day, with love and dedication. It means choosing, every day, to treat the other with kindness, to listen attentively, to be honest even when it is difficult, and to offer support without expectations.It is important to remember that no relationship is perfect, and we all, at times, may fail to show respect, maintain trust, or be fully reciprocal. But a strong relationship is one where both partners are willing to work together, to acknowledge their mistakes, and to do what they can to improve. It is a relationship where growth never stops because both know that the bond they share is precious and deserves to be cared for with attention.A relationship based on these values not only brings emotional well-being but becomes a true anchor of stability and strength in both partners' lives. It is a place where each person can feel secure, knowing the other is there not just out of love, but with deep respect for who they are.

Conclusion: The Art of Building Lasting Relationships Building relationships based on respect, trust, and reciprocity is a true art. It is a daily commitment made of small gestures, sincere words, and attentive listening. It is a journey of mutual discovery, where each partner learns not only to know the other but also to respect them, trust them, and build a balanced emotional exchange.Relationships like these are not only a source of joy and love but are also a place for personal growth. Through respect, trust, and reciprocity, we can learn to be ourselves in our most authentic form, knowing the other will accept, love, and support us. And in this safe space, we can finally flourish, building connections that not only accompany us through life but also transform us, making us better people.

Learning Assertiveness: Expressing Needs and Desires Without Depending on Others

Assertiveness is a subtle and valuable quality, positioned between passivity and aggressiveness, allowing us to express who we are in a clear and respectful way without self-neglect or overpowering others. It is the art of communicating our needs, desires, and boundaries while maintaining respect for others, but most importantly, for ourselves. Learning assertiveness means finding your inner voice, cultivating deep confidence in your worth, and opening yourself to more authentic and free relationships, without depending on recognition or approval from others.Being assertive does not mean raising your voice or imposing your will, nor does it mean conforming out of fear of displeasing others. Instead, it is the ability to assert oneself, to recognize your needs and desires as valid, and to communicate them in a respectful yet firm manner. It's a dialogue born from the awareness that our voice holds the same value as the other's, that we deserve space, listening, and consideration, and that we can live in relationships based on mutual respect without compromising who we are.

1 **The Difference Between Assertiveness, Passivity, and AggressivenessAssertiveness** is often misunderstood. Many people confuse it with aggressiveness, imagining that being assertive means being demanding or forceful. On the contrary, assertiveness lies in a delicate balance between passivity and aggressiveness, allowing us to be clear and direct without hurting or disrespecting others.

   ◦   **Passivity** occurs when, out of fear of conflict or a desire to please, we avoid expressing our needs or desires.

We give in, remain silent, allow our boundaries to be
ignored or violated, and end up feeling frustrated,
unheard, or worse, invisible.

- **Aggressiveness**, on the other hand, is the expression of
one's needs and desires in a dominating or forceful
way, without regard for the other person. In this
case, we impose our will without leaving room for
dialogue, fueling conflicts and tension.

Assertiveness, by contrast, is an act of balance and
authenticity. It means asserting one's needs clearly and
respectfully, finding solutions that take the other person into
account without yielding or attacking. Being assertive doesn't
mean imposing, but asking clearly while maintaining open and
respectful communication, where both can express their needs
without feeling threatened or at fault.

- **Reflection exercise on communication:** Reflect on a recent situation
where you wanted to express a need or desire but didn't.
Ask yourself, "Was I passive, or was I too aggressive?
How could I have expressed that need more assertively?"
This exercise will help you start identifying moments
where your communication could become more balanced.

2 **Recognizing and Validating Your Needs: The Foundation of
Assertiveness**To be assertive, the first step is learning to
recognize and validate your needs and desires. Often, we
put aside what we really want, fearing judgment,
rejection, or misunderstanding. However, to live
authentically and meaningfully, it is crucial to accept that
our needs are valid and worthy of being heard.Many
people grow up with the idea that putting others first is a
virtue, that self-sacrifice equates to kindness and
altruism. While generosity is a valuable quality, living in
constant self-sacrifice often means denying one's identity
and desires. Assertiveness is, first and foremost, an act of
self-care: it is the acknowledgment that we deserve to be
heard and respected, and that expressing what we want is
not selfish, but a gesture of respect toward
ourselves.Recognizing your needs means listening to your
emotions, understanding what makes you feel fulfilled,
calm, or uncomfortable. Only when we are aware of what

we truly want can we begin to communicate it with clarity and conviction.

- **Exercise for recognizing needs:** Each day, take a few minutes to reflect on what you need at that moment. It could be something emotional (like the need for affection or listening) or something practical (like the need for time alone). Write these reflections down to get used to recognizing and giving value to your needs.

3 **Communicating Clearly and Respectfully: The Art of Assertive Dialogue**Once you recognize your needs, the next step is to communicate them clearly and respectfully. This is the heart of assertiveness: being able to speak about yourself without fear and without accusing the other person. Often, the fear of causing conflict leads us to remain silent or not be entirely honest about what we feel. But assertiveness is founded on honesty—on communication that directly expresses what we want without manipulation or psychological games.Assertive communication follows some fundamental guidelines:

- **Speak about yourself:** Use "I" statements, such as "I feel," "I need," or "I want," rather than accusing the other person. This avoids putting them on the defensive and encourages a more open conversation.
- **Be specific:** Don't leave room for misunderstandings or ambiguity. Express clearly what you need or desire, avoiding vague language or insinuations. Saying "I'd like to spend more time together" is much more effective than "We never spend enough time together," which can sound like an accusation.
- **Be firm, but kind:** Assertiveness is not aggressiveness. You can express your needs firmly without being rude or overbearing. It's a balance between clarity and respect for the other person.
- **Listen to the other person:** Assertive communication is a dialogue, not a monologue. After expressing your needs, listen to what the other person has to say, welcoming their perspective without judgment.

- **Assertive communication exercise:** The next time you feel the need to express a desire or boundary, formulate your request starting with "I feel that..." or "I need...". Practice this phrase multiple times in front of a mirror until it flows naturally and confidently.

4 **Cultivating Self-Confidence: The Foundation of Assertiveness** Being assertive requires a good dose of self-confidence. When we don't truly believe in the value of our needs, we tend not to express them, or we do so insecurely, allowing others to ignore or overpower us. Assertiveness is born from a deep awareness of one's worth, from the conviction that what we feel and desire deserves to be respected, not only by those around us but, first and foremost, by ourselves. Cultivating self-confidence is not something achieved overnight; it's a process that takes time and dedication. Each time we choose to speak honestly, each time we express a need, we strengthen this confidence. The more we learn to communicate assertively, the more we realize that our voice matters, and that we can be respected without always having to conform to others. Self-confidence is also built through small acts of self-care. Every gesture of respect toward ourselves, whether it's taking time to rest, saying no when necessary, or asking for what we need, contributes to strengthening our self-esteem and making us feel more secure in relationships.

- **Self-esteem building exercise:** Each evening, reflect on a small gesture of respect you made toward yourself during the day. It could be something simple, like saying "no" to a commitment you didn't want or expressing a need. Write down these reflections and celebrate every small step toward greater self-confidence.

5 **Learning to Say "No" with Kindness and Firmness** Saying "no" is often one of the biggest challenges for those learning to be assertive. The fear of disappointing, being rejected, or judged can lead us to say yes when we don't really want to, sacrificing our needs for the sake of others. However, saying "no" is an act of self-protection, a way to respect our boundaries without feeling guilty. Learning to say "no" with kindness and firmness is a fundamental part of assertiveness. When we say "no," we are not rejecting the other person but simply affirming that we cannot meet their request at that moment. A "no" said with respect

and understanding can even strengthen the relationship because it shows we respect ourselves enough to be honest.

- **Saying "no" exercise:** Think of a recent situation where you said yes but wanted to say no. Imagine going back and responding differently, using phrases like, "I appreciate you asking, but I can't do it right now," or "I'd rather not commit at this time." Practice this dialogue, and the next time you feel the need to say no, do so with kindness and confidence.

Conclusion: Assertiveness as a Tool for Inner Freedom Learning assertiveness is a journey toward greater inner freedom. It means finding your voice, respecting your needs and desires, and living in more authentic and respectful relationships. Assertiveness is not a skill developed overnight, but an art cultivated over time, with patience and awareness. Through assertiveness, we learn that our worth does not depend on others' approval but on our ability to be true to ourselves. Expressing your needs and desires with clarity and respect is an act of self-love, allowing you to live with greater serenity and confidence in your relationships, knowing that you can be heard and respected without having to sacrifice or hide.

The Importance of Open and Honest Communication Communication is the soul of human relationships, the subtle and invisible thread that connects hearts, thoughts, and emotions. Through it, we build bridges between ourselves and others, revealing who we are, sharing dreams, worries, and joys. However, for communication to be truly nourishing and transformative, it must be open and honest, free from filters and masks that hide us. Open and sincere communication is the key to building authentic relationships, where each person can feel seen, heard, and understood in their uniqueness. Communicating in an open and honest way doesn't just mean talking, but opening the heart and mind to the other, without fear of judgment or rejection. It is an act of courage and vulnerability, requiring trust not only in others but also in ourselves. In this space of authentic communication, relationships become places of growth and deep intimacy, where it is possible to build bonds that withstand difficulties and misunderstandings.

1 **Communication as a Bridge Between Souls**Imagine two islands far apart, immersed in a vast and deep ocean. These islands represent people, each with their own inner world made of thoughts, emotions, stories, and desires. Communication is the bridge that connects these islands, allowing each person to share their world with the other. Without this bridge, each island remains isolated, unable to truly connect with the other.Communicating in an open and sincere way means allowing the other person to see what is inside of us, to enter our world without barriers. When we communicate openly, we offer the other the opportunity to understand us, to know what moves us, what scares us, and what we desire. At the same time, we open ourselves to listening to the other, allowing them to express their inner world without fear of being judged.This exchange creates a deep connection, a bond not only based on words but on the desire to share authenticity and truth. A relationship without open communication is like a garden without sunlight: it can survive, but it will never truly bloom.

2 **The Act of Speaking and the Act of Listening: A Necessary Balance**Open and honest communication is not only about expressing oneself but also about the ability to listen to the other. Speaking is an act of openness, but listening is an act of love. Often, in the rush of daily life, we forget how important it is to stop and truly listen to what the other has to say. Not distracted or formal listening, but deep listening, where we suspend our judgments, prejudices, and interpretations to embrace the other in all their complexity.Listening sincerely means making space for the other, allowing them to express themselves without interruptions, without feeling the need to immediately respond or find a solution. When we listen this way, we communicate to the other that we are there for them, that their inner world has value, and that we are ready to receive what they want to share, even if it's difficult or uncomfortable.This balance between speaking and listening is fundamental to building open communication. If we speak without listening, we impose our worldview,

missing the opportunity to understand the other. If we listen without expressing ourselves, we end up hiding, sacrificing our voice and needs. True open communication is a continuous flow between self-expression and listening to the other, a dialogue that enriches both.

- **Deep listening exercise:** In your next conversation, focus exclusively on listening. Don't interrupt, don't immediately think of a response, but stay present with the other person, listening not only to the words but also to the tone of voice, body language, and emotions that emerge.

3 **Vulnerability as the Key to Honest Communication** Expressing oneself openly and honestly requires vulnerability. This term is often misunderstood, associated with weakness, but in reality, vulnerability is one of the highest forms of courage. When we express ourselves sincerely, without masks or defenses, we reveal who we truly are, with all our insecurities, fears, and imperfections. This makes us vulnerable because opening up means risking being misunderstood, rejected, or not accepted. But it is through vulnerability that true intimacy is built. When we choose to be sincere, to express what we feel without filtering or censoring, we offer the other a precious gift: the chance to truly know us. In honest communication, there is no room for power plays or manipulative dynamics. There is only truth, manifested in words, gestures, and silences. Being vulnerable means saying, "I'm scared," "I don't know what to do," "I need you," without fearing judgment. This sincerity creates a space of mutual authenticity, where both partners can grow and support each other. When we show vulnerability, we allow the other to do the same, and this opens the door to deeper and more meaningful communication.

- **Vulnerability exercise:** Think of a conversation where you held back from saying what you truly felt. How could you have expressed your need or fear more honestly? The next time you find yourself in a similar situation, try to share what you feel, even if it's difficult. This will help you build more authentic relationships.

4 **Transforming Conflict Through Open Communication**Open and honest communication is also the most powerful tool for transforming conflicts into opportunities for growth. In any relationship, conflicts are inevitable: there will always be differences of opinion, misunderstandings, or moments of tension. But how we handle these conflicts determines the quality of the relationship.In a relationship where communication is not open, conflict can turn into a battlefield, where people either shut down defensively or attack to protect themselves. Emotions build up, remain unexpressed, and eventually explode destructively. Conversely, open communication allows conflicts to be handled constructively, turning them into opportunities to clarify needs, better understand the other, and strengthen the bond.When we communicate honestly during a conflict, we are not trying to win or be right but to understand and be understood. We express what we feel without accusing, listen to the other without interrupting, and seek a solution that considers both parties' needs. In this way, conflict becomes a dance of negotiation and compromise, where both partners can feel respected and heard.

- **Conflict communication exercise:** The next time you find yourself in a conflict, try expressing your feelings using "I feel..." statements instead of accusing or criticizing. This will change the tone of the conversation, opening a space for dialogue rather than for attack.

5 **Open Communication as the Foundation of Trust**At the heart of every healthy and lasting relationship is trust, and trust is born from open communication. When we know we can rely on the other to express what they feel and think without hiding anything, we feel more secure and free in the relationship. Honest communication builds a common ground of understanding and respect, on which deep and stable trust can grow.Conversely, when communication is fragmented, partial, or manipulated, trust begins to crumble. Unspoken words, withheld truths, and half-truths create distance between people, leaving room for misunderstandings, suspicions, and insecurities. To build trust, both parties must commit to being honest with each

other, even when the truth is difficult to say or hear.Open communication allows each person to feel secure in the relationship, knowing that there are no hidden secrets or repressed emotions that could explode unpredictably. In this space of trust, both partners can grow, knowing that their bond is based on truth, not on illusions or false appearances.

Conclusion: Open Communication as a Path to Freedom and Intimacy Open and honest communication is one of the highest forms of love and respect we can offer and receive in a relationship. Through it, we build deep bonds capable of withstanding life's challenges and enriching our lives. Communicating openly means living authentically, allowing ourselves and others to express freely, without fear, without masks, and without pretenses.In this space of sincere communication, true intimacy is found: a place where we can be entirely ourselves, knowing the other will listen, understand, and accept us for who we are. And in this space, relationships not only survive but thrive, nourishing both hearts with the power of truth and authentic connection.

How to Avoid Falling Back into Old Dependency Patterns

There is a fine thread that ties the past to the present, an invisible web that intertwines our experiences, our wounds, and our deepest desires. When we commit to change, to breaking free from old patterns of dependency, we may begin to feel the relief of freedom. But it is precisely in those moments of transition, as we venture into new territory, that the pull of the past becomes stronger. Old habits, familiar fears, and defense mechanisms often resurface like shadows, ready to make us fall back into what we know, into what once defined us.

Avoiding a relapse into these old dynamics requires awareness, determination, and a constant commitment to self-examination. It's an inner journey that is not accomplished once and for all, but must be traveled with patience and compassion. Every step forward requires us to pause and reflect on what held us back in the past, and how we can respond to ourselves and our relationships in new, healthier, and freer ways. It's a journey of healing, where we learn to recognize warning signs, strengthen our emotional autonomy, and create a space of love and respect within ourselves.

1. Awareness as a Tool for Freedom

The first key to avoiding falling back into old patterns of dependency is to develop a deep awareness of ourselves and our emotions. Often, dependency patterns are rooted in unconscious habits that make us seek in others what we cannot find within ourselves: approval, security, value. Without this awareness, it's easy to repeat the same patterns, as dependency mechanisms are like emotional traps that catch us when we are least vigilant.

Being aware means learning to recognize the warning signs: the excessive need for validation, the irrational fear of abandonment, the constant self-sacrifice to maintain the relationship. Awareness requires continuous inner observation, a constant dialogue with ourselves that helps us understand when we are falling into old patterns and how to correct our course.

To develop this awareness, it's important to take time to reflect on our past and present relationships. What patterns are recurring? Are there behaviors or emotions that seem to bring us back to a familiar but destructive place? This self-reflection work helps us prevent relapses and strengthens our ability to choose healthier, more balanced relationships.

Awareness Exercise: Every day, take a few minutes to reflect on a relationship or situation that matters to you. Ask yourself, "Am I acting in a healthy way, or am I falling into an old pattern?" Write down your thoughts and notice if any recurring patterns emerge. This practice will help you develop greater awareness of your emotional dynamics.

2. Learning to Manage the Fear of Loneliness

One of the central aspects of emotional dependency is the fear of loneliness. Often, dependency is rooted in the fear of being alone, in the terror of the emptiness that is felt when the other person is not present or does not meet our needs. This fear can lead us to do anything to maintain a relationship, even at the cost of our well-being and dignity.

Learning to manage loneliness is a fundamental part of the healing process. Being able to be alone doesn't mean isolating oneself, but developing a relationship with ourselves that allows us to feel complete and at peace even without the constant presence of another. It is in this space of solitude that we learn to cultivate our intrinsic value, to recognize that we do not need another to feel worthy of love and respect.

Managing loneliness requires a daily practice of self-compassion and self-care. Rather than fearing moments of solitude, we can see them as opportunities for growth, moments in which we can dedicate ourselves to what we love, explore our interests, and strengthen our emotional autonomy. The more we learn to be alone with ourselves, the less we feel the need to fill the void with a dependent relationship.

Mindful Solitude Exercise: Each week, set aside time to do something alone, without seeking external company. Whether it's a walk, a hobby, or simply a moment of reflection, embrace your solitude as a moment of connection with yourself. Write down the emotions you experience during these moments and observe how your relationship with loneliness changes over time.

3. Establishing Clear Boundaries and Respecting Them

Boundaries are essential to maintaining healthy relationships and avoiding a return to dependency patterns. Without clear boundaries, we risk losing ourselves in the other, sacrificing our needs and desires for fear of being abandoned. Boundaries are like a protective barrier that allows us to maintain our integrity, even within a relationship.

Establishing clear boundaries means knowing when to say no, when to ask for time and space for oneself, and when to communicate your needs without fear of rejection or conflict. But setting boundaries is not enough: we must also learn to respect them and have others respect them as well. Often, those who have experienced dependency dynamics tend to compromise their boundaries out of fear of losing the relationship, but it is precisely by respecting boundaries that we can build relationships based on mutual respect.

Boundary-Setting Exercise: Take a moment to reflect on the boundaries you feel you need to set in your relationships. It could be the need for more personal space, time for yourself, or greater emotional autonomy. Write down these boundaries and commit to respecting them, even if it may be difficult at first.

4. Strengthening Self-Esteem and Self-Love

At the root of emotional dependency is often a lack of self-esteem. When we don't feel enough, we tend to seek validation from others. But this makes us vulnerable to dependency, as our sense of self depends on external factors. Strengthening self-confidence and cultivating self-love is one of the most powerful steps in avoiding falling back into old patterns of dependency.

Self-esteem doesn't arise out of nowhere, but is built through small acts of self-respect, day by day. Every time we choose to treat ourselves with kindness, acknowledge our successes, or take care of our emotional needs, we are strengthening our self-esteem. This allows us to enter relationships from a place of strength and fullness, without depending on others to feel complete.

Self-love is the foundation on which healthy relationships are built. When we learn to love ourselves, we will no longer accept relationships that harm us, and we will be less inclined to sacrifice ourselves to gain love or approval from others.

Self-Esteem Building Exercise: Each day, take a moment to reflect on something positive you've done or an aspect of yourself that you appreciate. Write these reflections in a journal and read them again in moments when you feel insecure or vulnerable. This will help you develop greater confidence in yourself.

5. Seeking External Support: The Strength of Healthy Relationships

Breaking free from old dependency patterns is a process that requires support. While inner work is essential, it is equally important to have a network of healthy, supportive relationships around you. This can include friends, family, but also the support of a therapist or a support group. Talking to people who understand our journey and offer empathetic listening can make a difference in difficult times.

Healthy relationships offer us a mirror through which we can see ourselves more clearly, without distortions or manipulations. Having people who respect, support, and encourage us to grow strengthens our ability to maintain emotional autonomy and avoid falling back into old patterns.

Relational Support Exercise: Identify the people in your life who offer you positive and nurturing support. Dedicate time to cultivating these relationships, expressing gratitude for their support. If you feel the need for further help, consider seeking a therapist or support group that can guide you in your healing journey.

Conclusion: A Journey Toward Freedom and Emotional Autonomy

Avoiding falling back into old dependency patterns is an ongoing process, a journey of awareness, self-care, and conscious choice. Each step toward emotional freedom brings us closer to authentic relationships, based on respect, reciprocity, and love. When we learn to recognize our needs, manage the fear of loneliness, and strengthen our self-esteem, we become capable of building a more balanced and fulfilling relational life.

In this journey, there are no shortcuts, but every small victory, every act of self-care, brings us closer to a life where we can love and be loved without depending on others for our sense of completeness. It is a path toward emotional freedom, where we can finally be who we are, without fear, without needing external validation, but grounded in a deep trust in ourselves and our worth.

Part 5: Living Love in a Healthy and Autonomous Way Chapter 13

Self-Love

What It Means to Love Yourself: Acceptance and Self-Compassion

Loving yourself is a revolutionary act, one of the most profound and transformative gestures we can make for our well-being and inner life. It is not an act of selfishness, as is often misunderstood, but an act of radical acceptance and self-compassion that allows us to recognize ourselves as worthy of love, respect, and care, without having to prove anything to anyone, not even to ourselves. It is the art of embracing our humanity, with all its imperfections, weaknesses, and contradictions, and finding peace in being exactly who we are.

Loving yourself is a silent revolution, because in a world that constantly pushes us to improve, to be stronger, more perfect, more successful, choosing to accept and love who we are, without conditions, becomes an act of profound inner freedom. It is an invitation to treat ourselves with the same kindness and care we reserve for the people we love, to recognize that we are worthy of love despite our mistakes and our vulnerabilities — in fact, because of them.

1. Self-Acceptance: Embracing Your Humanity

Self-love begins with acceptance. Accepting yourself means recognizing who you are, both good and bad, without trying to hide the parts of yourself that you find uncomfortable, imperfect, or unworthy. It's about looking in the mirror and saying, "I am enough, just as I am." Not because we are perfect, but because we are whole in our complexity. Self-acceptance is not resignation, nor is it a passive act, but rather a gesture of deep wisdom that invites us to stop fighting against ourselves.

Many of us spend a large part of our lives trying to change or improve aspects of ourselves that we consider inadequate. We constantly compare ourselves to others, to an ideal of perfection that always seems out of reach, and in the constant chase to be different, we forget to recognize and accept who we really are. Acceptance, on the other hand, invites us to make peace with our authentic selves, to embrace not only our successes but also our failures, not only our strengths but also our vulnerabilities.

Accepting yourself means looking at your shadows, the parts of yourself you hide, and welcoming them with kindness. It means stopping self-judgment, ceasing to criticize yourself, and refraining from feeling defective for not being perfect. It's the art of saying, "It's okay. I'm a human being, and that's enough."

Acceptance Exercise: Every morning, take a few minutes to stand in front of the mirror. Look yourself in the eyes and say aloud, "I accept myself for who I am, with my strengths and my weaknesses." Notice the feelings that arise and try to make peace with the parts of yourself you tend to judge. This daily practice will help you ground self-acceptance in your everyday life.

2. Self-Compassion: Treating Yourself with Kindness

Acceptance is the first step in loving yourself, but to cultivate deep and lasting love, it is essential to develop self-compassion. Compassion, in its truest form, is the act of seeing someone's suffering and wanting to alleviate it. Self-compassion means applying this kindness to ourselves, especially in times of difficulty, error, or failure. It means acknowledging our pain and offering ourselves comfort and understanding instead of judgment and criticism.

Many people, when they make a mistake or go through a difficult time, treat themselves with a harshness and severity they would never show to a friend. We blame ourselves, criticize ourselves, and end up believing that we are not good enough or worthy of love. Self-compassion invites us to completely change our inner dialogue, replacing criticism with words of kindness and care.

Self-compassion doesn't mean justifying our mistakes or avoiding responsibility, but rather learning to forgive ourselves and treat ourselves with the same gentleness we offer those we love. It means saying, "It's okay to make mistakes, it's okay not to be perfect. I'm a human being, and I deserve love even in my darkest moments."

Being self-compassionate means recognizing that all of us, as human beings, experience moments of suffering and failure, and it is precisely in those moments that we need tenderness, support, and acceptance the most.

Self-Compassion Exercise: Every time you catch yourself criticizing or judging yourself harshly, stop and take a deep breath. Imagine speaking to yourself as you would to a dear friend, using words of comfort and encouragement. Try saying, "I'm doing my best, and that's okay." This simple gesture can profoundly change the way you relate to yourself.

3. Stop Seeking Perfection: Being Enough Just as You Are

We live in a society that constantly bombards us with images of perfection: perfect bodies, perfect lives, perfect successes. This creates an illusion that pushes us to believe that in order to be loved, accepted, or respected, we must meet these impossible standards. But self-love begins when we learn to let go of perfection and recognize that we are already enough, exactly as we are.

Perfection is a mirage, an idea that shifts and changes every time we think we've reached it. In chasing it, we lose sight of the beauty in our imperfection, our uniqueness, which is what makes us human and connected to others. Loving yourself means recognizing that completeness is not found in perfection, but in accepting all parts of ourselves, even those that seem flawed or incomplete.

Learning to stop seeking perfection is an act of liberation. It allows us to live with more lightness, to appreciate who we are without the constant weight of judgment or the fear of failure. It is an act of trust in ourselves, in our ability to be worthy of love precisely because of our authenticity.

Liberation from Perfection Exercise: Every time you catch yourself striving for perfection in some area of your life, stop and ask yourself, "Why do I want to be perfect in this? What am I trying to prove or achieve?" Recognize that perfection is not necessary to be loved or accepted, and make a small act of kindness toward yourself by accepting imperfection as a natural part of life.

4. Cultivating Positive Self-Talk: Speaking to Yourself with Love

The way we talk to ourselves has a profound impact on our sense of worth and our ability to love who we are. Often, without even realizing it, we carry on an inner dialogue filled with negativity, criticism, and judgment. We tell ourselves we're not good enough, that we don't deserve love, that we need to do more, be more. But our inner dialogue is one of the keys to building a healthy, loving relationship with ourselves.

Learning to speak to yourself with love means replacing negative talk with words of encouragement, trust, and affection. It means becoming your greatest ally, rather than your harshest critic. Start with small changes: every time you notice a criticism, try turning it into a word of encouragement. If you think, "I'm not good enough," turn it into, "I'm doing my best, and that's enough."

Positive self-talk is not a form of self-deception, but a conscious choice to treat ourselves with kindness and compassion. It helps create a fertile ground for self-love, where we can grow, make mistakes, and learn without harshly judging ourselves.

Positive Self-Talk Exercise: Every evening before bed, reflect on one positive thing you did during the day, even if it was small. Speak words of appreciation to yourself and acknowledge your efforts. This will help you cultivate a kinder inner dialogue and nurture self-love.

5. Self-Love as the Foundation of Healthy Relationships

Loving yourself not only allows you to live with greater serenity and self-esteem, but it also becomes the foundation for building healthy and fulfilling relationships. When we learn to respect and accept ourselves, we no longer feel the need to seek validation of our worth from others. We enter relationships from a place of wholeness, not lack, knowing that we deserve love and respect without having to sacrifice or conform to receive it.

Self-love gives us the courage to set healthy boundaries, to say "no" when necessary, and to express our needs without fear of rejection. It allows us to live relationships more authentically, without depending on the other to feel complete. When we love ourselves, we become capable of giving love more genuinely because we are no longer trying to fill a void, but to share our fullness.

Conclusion: Loving Yourself as an Act of Freedom and Compassion

Loving yourself is the greatest act of freedom we can undertake. It means freeing ourselves from the expectations, criticisms, and judgments we have internalized, to embrace our deepest truth. Through acceptance and self-compassion, we learn to recognize our intrinsic worth, to treat ourselves kindly even in difficult times, and to build a life based on love, respect, and self-care.

In this space of self-love, we find the strength to face life with serenity, to build healthier and more authentic relationships, and to live fully, knowing that we deserve all the good we can offer ourselves. Self-love is a journey, not a destination, but every step along this path brings us closer to our essence, our truth, and the full realization of who we are.

Self-Care Practices: Meditation, Physical Activity, and Hobbies

Self-care is a delicate art, a daily act of love for the mind, body, and spirit. In a world that moves relentlessly, urging us to do, achieve, and produce, taking care of ourselves becomes an act of quiet rebellion. It is not a superficial or selfish gesture, but a profound commitment to our inner well-being and balanced flourishing. Self-care means creating a sacred space in our lives where we can listen to our needs, nurture what feeds our soul, and let go of what no longer serves us.

Self-care practices take many forms: from meditation, which reconnects us to our inner core, to physical activity, which grounds us in the body and awakens its vitality, and hobbies, which provide space for our spirit to express itself freely. Each of these practices is an invitation to return home, to reconnect with ourselves, and to discover a new depth in our existence.

1. Meditation: A Journey Back to Yourself

Meditation is one of the oldest and most powerful self-care tools. It is a silent journey that takes us deep into our inner being, beyond the noise of the mind, beyond daily anxieties, to touch that place of peace that always exists within us. Meditating doesn't necessarily mean sitting in silence for hours; it is more an act of presence, an intimate encounter with the here and now, which allows us to observe what is happening inside and outside of us without judgment.

In meditation, we learn to slow down, make space for the breath, and let thoughts drift away like clouds in the sky. It is a moment of grounding where we remind ourselves that, even in the chaos of life, there is an unshakable core within us, a place of deep calm to which we can always return. Meditation allows us to build a more intimate relationship with our emotions, to acknowledge them without being overwhelmed, and to cultivate a clearer and more serene mind.

Meditation is not only a spiritual practice but also a powerful form of caring for our mental well-being. It reduces stress, relieves anxiety, and allows us to face life with greater clarity and centeredness. Every time we take time to meditate, we are making a loving gesture toward ourselves, creating a sacred space for listening and regeneration.

Daily Meditation Exercise: Every day, dedicate 5–10 minutes to meditation. Sit in a quiet place, close your eyes, and focus on your breath. Observe the air entering and leaving your body without trying to control it. If thoughts arise, simply observe them and let them pass, like leaves carried by a stream. This simple practice will help you cultivate presence and reduce daily stress.

2. Physical Activity: Awakening the Body and Vitality

Physical activity is another essential form of self-care, a way to reconnect with your body, listen to it, and awaken its vitality. We live in a time where the mind often prevails over the body, leaving us disconnected from its needs and natural rhythms. But the body is our temple, the vehicle that allows us to live and experience the world, and it deserves to be treated with care and respect.

Physical activity is not just about physical fitness or aesthetics; it is a way to release blocked energy, to let vitality flow through every cell of our being. When we move—whether through dancing, yoga, running, or simply walking—we give our body permission to express itself, to release accumulated tension, and to regain its natural state of balance.

Physical movement has a profound impact not only on the body but also on the mind. It releases endorphins, the so-called happiness hormones, reduces stress, and improves mood. It is an act of love toward ourselves, a way of caring for our body not as an object to be improved but as an integral part of our overall well-being.

Mindful Physical Activity Exercise: Every day, set aside at least 20 minutes for physical activity that you enjoy. It could be an outdoor run, a yoga session, a walk in nature, or a liberating dance at home. Listen to your body as it moves, focus on how it feels, and enjoy the sense of liberation and vitality that movement gives you.

3. Hobbies: The Sacred Space for Self-Expression

Hobbies are one of the most often overlooked aspects of self-care, but they are a key element in cultivating our inner joy. In a world that constantly pushes us toward productivity, finding time for personal interests may seem like a luxury, but it is actually an essential need for our creativity and emotional well-being.

A hobby is more than just a pastime; it is a sacred space where we can express ourselves freely, without expectations or external pressures. Whether it's writing, painting, playing a musical instrument, cooking, gardening, or any other activity that excites us, hobbies allow us to disconnect from daily worries and enter a state of creative flow. In this space, time seems to dissolve, and we are fully present in the activity, with a light mind and an open heart.

Cultivating a hobby is an act of nourishing the soul because it allows us to explore our creativity and connect with what brings us joy. No matter how busy or stressed we are, finding time for the activities we are passionate about is a way of reminding ourselves that life is also about pleasure, discovery, and lightness.

Hobby Exploration Exercise: If you haven't found a hobby that excites you yet, take some time to explore new activities. Try something new every week: a painting class, a cooking lesson, a photography walk. Notice what makes you feel most alive and cultivate that activity as an essential part of your self-care.

4. The Ritual of Daily Care: A Commitment to Yourself

Self-care is not a luxury or something reserved for moments of crisis, but a daily ritual that helps us maintain balance in life. Like a garden that needs to be watered every day, so do our body, mind, and spirit need regular attention and care. Taking care of ourselves means making a pact of love with ourselves, where we commit to dedicating time and space to our well-being, despite the endless external demands.

Every self-care practice, whether it's meditation, physical activity, or a hobby, is an act of self-renewal. It's a way of reminding ourselves that we deserve time, attention, and love. It doesn't matter how brief the moments we manage to dedicate to these practices; what matters is the consistency and intention with which we carry them out. It's the message we send to ourselves every time we choose to care for ourselves: "I am important. My well-being is a priority."

Daily Care Exercise: Create a small daily care ritual that includes at least one self-care practice. It could be a brief morning meditation, an afternoon walk, or half an hour dedicated to your favorite hobby. Write this commitment on a piece of paper and keep it visible as a reminder that every day you deserve to dedicate a moment to self-care and attention.

Conclusion: The Power of Self-Care for a Full and Meaningful Life

Self-care is a form of love and respect for ourselves. It is the recognition that we cannot give to the world and others unless we first nourish our inner being. Through meditation, physical activity, and hobbies, we learn to care for ourselves in a holistic way: body, mind, and spirit. These practices not only improve our physical and mental well-being but also allow us to live more presently, with a sense of fulfillment and satisfaction that goes beyond doing and producing.

In this fast-paced, overstimulated world, self-care becomes an act of grounding and returning home, an inner journey that brings us back to our center, where we can rediscover our truth and essence. It is a journey that invites us to slow down, breathe, and remember that life is not just a race and competition, but also joy, creativity, and peace.

Through self-care, we can rediscover the beauty of living in harmony with ourselves, with others, and with the world around us.

Learning to Be Your Own Emotional Support

Being your own emotional support is a subtle art, a form of inner strength that doesn't reveal itself in toughness, but in the ability to offer yourself tenderness and understanding during difficult moments. In a world where we often seek comfort and security from external sources, learning to be your own emotional support represents an act of radical autonomy and deep maturity. It means developing a relationship of trust with yourself, where you know you can face emotional storms with courage and serenity, without depending exclusively on others for your inner balance.

Becoming your own emotional support doesn't imply isolating yourself or rejecting external support; rather, it means learning to rely on yourself first and foremost. It is an act of deep self-compassion, recognizing that even in moments of vulnerability, we have within us the resources to heal, to calm ourselves, and to regain our center. This ability makes us more resilient, more confident in who we are, and allows us to live relationships with greater freedom, without the constant fear of being abandoned or misunderstood.

1. Building an Intimate Relationship with Yourself

The first step to becoming your own emotional support is to develop an intimate and authentic relationship with yourself. Often, we spend much of our lives seeking approval and comfort from others, forgetting to listen to how we truly feel and to embrace what we experience. But to be our greatest ally, we must learn to deeply know ourselves, to explore our emotional world without fear, without fleeing from our emotions.

This intimate relationship with yourself requires presence and self-listening. In difficult moments, instead of immediately seeking someone to lift us up, we can pause and ask ourselves: "What am I feeling? What do I really need right now?" This act of self-reflection allows us to connect with our authentic self, to understand our emotions without judging them, and to respond with kindness.

The relationship we build with ourselves is the most important one of our lives because it's the only one that lasts forever. Learning to console and support ourselves during vulnerable moments is an act of profound love for oneself. It reminds us that we are never truly alone, because within us exists a strength capable of offering support and understanding, even in the most difficult times.

Self-Listening Exercise: Every time you feel overwhelmed or emotionally vulnerable, take some time to be with yourself. Close your eyes, take a deep breath, and ask yourself: "What am I feeling right now? What do I need to hear from myself?" Write your responses in a journal, and practice self-reflection daily to develop a deeper connection with your emotional world.

2. Developing Self-Compassion: Being Your Own Best Friend

Being your own emotional support also means learning to treat yourself with self-compassion, especially in moments of error or failure. Too often, when we find ourselves struggling, our immediate reaction is to criticize ourselves, to feel inadequate, or to think we're not enough. But harshness toward ourselves never leads to healing; on the contrary, it isolates us even more and sinks us deeper into pain.

Self-compassion is the art of being your own best friend. It's the ability to offer ourselves the same comfort, love, and understanding we would reserve for a loved one. It means recognizing that suffering is part of being human and that we don't need to be perfect to deserve kindness and care.

When we practice self-compassion, we learn to support our difficult emotions with gentleness. Instead of judging ourselves for what we feel, we welcome our emotions as we would a frightened child: with calm, patience, and tenderness. This practice helps us develop greater emotional resilience because we know that, no matter what happens, we can always count on our own love and care.

Self-Compassion Exercise: Every time you feel self-judgment creeping in, try to change your inner dialogue. Ask yourself: "How would I speak to a friend who feels this way?" Then, say those same comforting words to yourself, remembering that you deserve the same love and kindness.

3. Taking Responsibility for Your Emotions

Being your own emotional support also means taking responsibility for your emotions. Instead of looking outside for someone to resolve our discomfort or make us feel better, we learn to care for our emotions with awareness and autonomy. This doesn't mean rejecting the support of others, but recognizing that, ultimately, we are the guardians of our inner well-being.

When we take responsibility for our emotions, we stop projecting our expectations of comfort and security onto others. We understand that our emotions belong to us and that we have the power to influence how we manage and respond to them. This allows us to avoid emotional dependence on others and develop greater inner stability.

Caring for your emotions also means learning to regulate them in healthy ways. When we feel overwhelmed by anger, fear, or sadness, we can learn to observe these emotions without reacting immediately, allowing them to express themselves without being consumed by them. This process helps us develop greater emotional autonomy and build a healthier relationship with our inner world.

Emotional Responsibility Exercise: Every time you experience a strong emotion, pause for a moment and observe how you feel. Ask yourself: "This emotion belongs to me. How can I take care of it without projecting it onto others?" This exercise will help you develop greater awareness and manage your emotions with responsibility.

4. Cultivating Self-Trust: Believing in Your Inner Strength

One of the most important aspects of being your own emotional support is developing deep self-trust. It means believing that, no matter what happens, we have the inner strength to face life's challenges. This trust doesn't stem from the illusion of invulnerability but from the awareness that we are capable of facing difficulties with resilience and wisdom.

Self-trust is built through small acts of daily courage. Every time we choose to face a difficult situation calmly, every time we care for our emotions without seeking refuge externally, we are strengthening our inner trust. The more we learn to support ourselves, the more we realize that we are capable of handling life in all its complexity.

Self-trust allows us to live with greater serenity, knowing that even in tough times, we can rely on our inner strength. We are no longer at the mercy of external circumstances or the expectations of others, but rooted in a deep trust in our worth and our capacity to heal.

Self-Trust Building Exercise: Every evening, reflect on a challenge you faced during the day and how you managed to overcome it. Acknowledge your successes, no matter how small, and celebrate the fact that you faced the situation with strength and determination. This will help you build greater self-trust.

5. Creating Emotional Care Rituals

To become your own emotional support, it is important to create emotional care rituals that help us maintain balance and inner well-being. These rituals can be simple daily gestures, like taking time for meditation, physical exercise, or journaling. The important thing is that they are practices that allow us to connect with ourselves and nurture our inner world.

Emotional care rituals offer us a safe space where we can relax, reflect, and rejuvenate. They are moments dedicated solely to us, where we can listen to our emotions and respond to them with kindness. Creating these rituals helps remind us every day that we are our greatest ally and that we deserve time, attention, and care.

Emotional Care Ritual Exercise: Create an emotional care ritual that you can practice every day. It could be a brief morning meditation, a relaxing evening bath, or a few minutes of journaling where you explore your emotions. Commit to practicing this ritual consistently and lovingly, knowing that it is an act of deep respect for yourself.

Conclusion: The Freedom of Being Your Own Emotional Support

Learning to be your own emotional support is a journey toward freedom and inner autonomy. It is a path that leads us to develop a relationship of trust with ourselves, to cultivate self-compassion, and to take responsibility for our emotions. Along this path, we discover that strength is not found in seeking refuge in others, but in building a safe haven within ourselves, where we can always return for comfort, understanding, and love.

Becoming your own emotional support doesn't mean shutting yourself off from others but rather living relationships with greater fullness and authenticity, without depending on others for your well-being. It is a journey toward emotional autonomy, where we learn to navigate life's storms with calm and centeredness, knowing that, no matter what happens, we can count on ourselves.

The Role of Gratitude and Self-Forgiveness

Gratitude and forgiveness are two silent yet powerful forces capable of transforming our inner world, healing invisible wounds, and renewing our relationship with ourselves. When we learn to practice gratitude and forgiveness toward ourselves, we embark on a path of liberation and deep acceptance that allows us to live with greater lightness and authenticity. In a society that constantly pushes us to be stronger, more perfect, more successful, rediscovering the beauty of gratitude and forgiveness represents an act of inner revolution.

Loving oneself is not a linear process; it's a path filled with steps forward and backward, successes and mistakes. But it is through the conscious practice of gratitude and forgiveness that we can learn to embrace our authentic selves, accepting not only our light but also our shadows. Gratitude and forgiveness become two beacons guiding us through the darkness of our uncertainties and imperfections, illuminating the way toward a more mature, complete, and unconditional self-love.

1. Gratitude Towards Yourself: Cultivating Inner Abundance

Often, when we think of gratitude, we imagine directing it outward: thanking the people around us, fortunate events, or life's opportunities. But how often do we stop to thank ourselves? Gratitude toward oneself is rare but extraordinarily powerful. It is the ability to recognize the value of our efforts, to appreciate our resilience, growth, and learning despite difficulties.

Being grateful toward yourself means seeing yourself with more compassionate eyes, recognizing that even in tough moments, you are doing your best. It's an act of self-acknowledgment, where you don't wait for others to validate your worth, but you do it yourself. When we pause to thank ourselves for who we are, what we have done, and our progress, we sow seeds of joy and inner peace in our hearts.

Gratitude toward oneself is a way to nurture our soul, reminding us that we are not just our mistakes or imperfections but also our successes, our small daily victories, and our ability to face challenges with courage. When we cultivate this gratitude, we begin to see our life not as an endless race toward unreachable improvement, but as a journey already full of riches that deserve to be celebrated.

Self-Gratitude Exercise: Every evening before bed, take a few minutes to reflect on three things you can be grateful for about yourself. It could be a small gesture you made, a decision you took, or simply the fact that you were there for yourself during the day. Write these reflections in a journal and reread them whenever you need to be reminded of your worth.

2. Forgiveness Towards Yourself: Releasing the Weight of Self-Judgment

If gratitude teaches us to see the abundance within us, forgiveness is the act that allows us to release the weight we carry in our hearts. Often, we are much more ready to forgive others than we are to forgive ourselves. We hold on to our mistakes and failures, reliving them as if they were scars that can never heal. But true forgiveness begins within: it is an act of liberation, a way to make peace with our past, with the choices we wish we hadn't made, with the words we wish we hadn't said.

Forgiving oneself is difficult because we often feel we must atone for our mistakes, as if we don't deserve to be free from the pain we inflict on ourselves. But forgiveness is not a way of denying responsibility or justifying our mistakes. On the contrary, it is an act of radical compassion: we acknowledge what happened, we learn from it, and then we choose not to let our past continue to define us. Forgiveness is the key that frees us from the chains of self-judgment and allows us to look toward the future with brighter, more confident eyes.

When we forgive ourselves, we are telling ourselves that we are human, that we are imperfect, and that this is okay. We are accepting that mistakes are part of our journey and that we don't need to punish ourselves for falling. The more we learn to forgive ourselves, the easier it becomes to live lightly, without the constant weight of unrealistic expectations we place on ourselves.

Self-Forgiveness Exercise: Think of a mistake or failure from your past that still haunts you. Take a few minutes to reflect on what happened and then say, either out loud or to yourself, these words: "I forgive myself for this mistake. I did my best with the resources I had at the time, and now I choose to move forward with lightness." Repeat this exercise whenever you feel the weight of self-judgment.

3. Gratitude and Forgiveness as Healing Tools

Gratitude and forgiveness are two sides of the same coin: both help heal our relationship with ourselves. Gratitude teaches us to celebrate what is already present in our lives, to see the beauty in small things, to recognize our achievements and not take them for granted. Forgiveness, on the other hand, allows us to let go of what weighs us down, freeing ourselves from regrets and remorse, and embracing a lighter, more serene life.

When we learn to combine gratitude and forgiveness, we create a sacred space within ourselves, where we can dwell in peace, without the anxiety of having to be perfect or better. In this space, we allow ourselves to be fully human, with all our contradictions and imperfections. Here, we are safe from external judgment, and most importantly, from our own.

Gratitude and forgiveness work together to create emotional balance: gratitude grounds us in the present, while forgiveness frees us from the past. Together, they allow us to live a fuller, more authentic life, where we can love ourselves for who we are, without waiting for something to change or improve.

Gratitude and Forgiveness Exercise: Every week, take a moment to reflect on both what you are grateful for about yourself and what you feel the need to forgive yourself for. Write these reflections down and, if you wish, create a small ritual of release, such as symbolically burning a piece of paper with what you want to let go. This will help you create a routine of emotional healing and personal growth.

4. The Transformative Power of Forgiveness and Gratitude in Daily Life

When gratitude and forgiveness become integral parts of our daily lives, we begin to notice a profound shift in how we relate not only to ourselves but also to others. Gratitude teaches us to see the good, even in difficult moments, to find light even in the darkest situations. Forgiveness allows us to navigate relationships with greater openness, knowing that we don't need to be perfect, nor do we need to wait for others to be.

Gratitude makes us appreciate the beauty of life, while forgiveness frees us from the chains of resentment and guilt. These two tools offer us a broader and more compassionate perspective on our path, reminding us that life is full of ups and downs, successes and failures, and that at any moment, we can choose to renew our relationship with ourselves and the world.

Daily Transformation Exercise: Each morning, before starting the day, think of one aspect of yourself for which you can be grateful and one aspect you wish to forgive. Carry these thoughts with you throughout the day, and observe them as anchors that bring you back to the present moment and serenity.

Conclusion: The Journey to Self-Love Through Gratitude and Forgiveness

Gratitude and forgiveness are the pillars on which deep and lasting self-love is built. They are the tools that allow us to free ourselves from impossible expectations, to embrace our imperfection, and to cherish the beauty of being human. When we learn to practice gratitude toward ourselves, we realize how abundant we already are, how much value we bring to the world, even without needing to be different from who we are.

Forgiveness, on the other hand, offers us the opportunity to let go of the weight of the past, to free ourselves from the yoke of judgment, and to walk through life with greater lightness and freedom. Together, gratitude and forgiveness teach us that we don't need to be perfect to deserve love. We are already whole, already worthy, just as we are.

On this journey of self-love, gratitude and forgiveness become lifelong companions, guides that constantly bring us back to our hearts, reminding us that, in the end, everything we seek outside can be found within. And that true love always begins here—with a "thank you" and a "I forgive you" directed toward ourselves.

Part 5: Living Love in a Healthy and Autonomous Way Chapter 14

Relationships and Healthy Love

How to Recognize a Healthy and Fulfilling Relationship

A healthy and fulfilling relationship is like a flourishing garden: it requires time, care, and the right combination of elements to thrive. It's a sacred space where two people can grow together, support each other through tough times, and celebrate moments of joy. Unlike toxic relationships, which drain energy and create disconnection, a healthy relationship nourishes the soul, offering fertile ground where both partners can blossom. It is a place of safety and respect, where mutual trust and open communication form the foundation of the bond.

Recognizing a healthy relationship means being able to identify subtle yet profound signs of balance, reciprocity, and authenticity. In a world where the idea of love is often idealized or distorted, learning to identify a relationship that truly enriches us is essential for our emotional and spiritual well-being.

1. Mutual Trust: The Foundation of Every Healthy Relationship

A healthy relationship is first and foremost built on mutual trust. Trust is like the lifeblood of a plant: without it, the bond dries up, cracks, and breaks. In a relationship based on trust, both partners know they can rely on each other without fear or suspicion. It is the certainty that the other will be there in times of need, that they won't betray or hide the truth. Trust creates a space of emotional security where each person can open up, be vulnerable, and share their deepest emotions without fear of being judged or hurt.

When trust is present, there is no need to control or doubt because both partners care about each other's well-being. Trust is built over time through small and large acts of honesty, integrity, and consistency. It is an essential pillar for creating a stable relationship where love is not based on illusions or unrealistic expectations, but on the awareness that, no matter what happens, there is mutual respect that never falters.

Sign of Trust: In a healthy relationship, you feel free to be yourself without fear of being judged or abandoned. You know that the other person respects you and honors your boundaries, and that you can openly discuss anything without damaging the trust between you.

2. Respect: The Key to Reciprocity

Respect is the foundation of every fulfilling relationship. It allows two people to recognize and value each other's differences without trying to change or manipulate the other. In a healthy relationship, respect is shown through the care and consideration both partners give to each other's needs, feelings, and boundaries. There is no room for devaluation, harsh words, or controlling behaviors. Respect is nurtured through active listening, constructive dialogue, and genuine attention toward the other.

In a healthy relationship, respect is not limited to moments of calm but emerges even during conflicts. Discussions are approached with kindness and maturity, avoiding insults or manipulative tactics. The partners know they may not agree on everything, but they are committed to treating each other with dignity. Mutual respect allows the relationship to deepen, creating a space where both can be authentic and vulnerable.

Sign of Respect: In a healthy relationship, your thoughts, feelings, and desires are listened to and respected. Even when there are disagreements, your partner does not belittle you or try to impose their views but listens and seeks a compromise that honors both of you.

3. Open and Honest Communication: The Heart of the Relationship

In a healthy relationship, communication is like the blood that flows, nourishing every part of the bond. It is through open and honest communication that partners can share their thoughts, emotions, and desires without fear of being misunderstood or ignored. The ability to speak honestly about what one feels, even when it's difficult, is what distinguishes a healthy relationship from a superficial or dysfunctional one.

Open communication is not just about expressing one's needs but also about the ability to listen to the other empathetically and respectfully. It's not just about talking but about creating a dialogue space where both partners can feel understood and welcomed. In a healthy relationship, there are no forced silences or unspoken words that create distance. Instead, the partners are willing to confront issues, solve problems, and grow together through clear and respectful communication.

Sign of Good Communication: In a healthy relationship, you feel free to express your thoughts and feelings without fearing excessive or punitive reactions. You know the other will listen to you with respect, even when there are difficulties, and that together you will find a solution.

4. Reciprocity: The Natural Flow of Giving and Receiving

One of the fundamental characteristics of a healthy and fulfilling relationship is reciprocity. In this type of bond, giving and receiving flow naturally and are balanced. Neither partner feels compelled to sacrifice themselves to maintain the relationship because both contribute with generosity and affection without expecting anything in return. Reciprocity is not only measured in practical acts but also in emotional support, listening, and respecting each other's time and needs.

Reciprocity creates a balance that prevents power dynamics or dependency from forming. When both partners feel valued and supported, the relationship becomes a space of mutual nourishment, where each can give their best without fear of being exploited or ignored. This type of relationship is based on a deep alliance, where love is not a competition or a struggle for control but a mutual exchange that enriches both.

Sign of Reciprocity: In a healthy relationship, you feel supported and valued as much as you offer your support to the other. You don't feel like you have to give more than you receive, and there is a natural balance between the times when you care for the other and the times when they care for you.

5. The Freedom to Be Yourself: A Refuge of Authenticity

A healthy relationship doesn't require you to change or conform to an ideal to be loved. Instead, it is a space where each person can fully be themselves, with all their imperfections and vulnerabilities. In this type of relationship, there are no masks or facades to maintain because both partners love and respect each other for who they truly are. The relationship becomes a refuge of authenticity, a place where one can be vulnerable without fear of being judged or rejected.

The freedom to be yourself in a healthy relationship is what allows the bond to evolve over time. When both people can grow and change without fear of losing the other's love or acceptance, the relationship becomes a flourishing garden, where individual growth also enriches the couple's connection.

Sign of Authenticity: In a healthy relationship, you don't feel obligated to hide parts of yourself out of fear of being judged or rejected. You can be vulnerable, talk about your dreams and fears, and know that your partner will welcome you with love and understanding without trying to change you.

6. Mutual Support: Growing Together on Life's Journey

In a healthy relationship, partners are not just life companions but allies who support each other in their personal growth. Each person wants the best for the other and is committed to being a source of encouragement and inspiration. There are no power struggles, jealousy, or attempts to undermine the other's success—just a genuine desire to see the other flourish.

Mutual support is shown in times of difficulty when life presents challenges and obstacles. In a healthy relationship, partners help each other, lift each other during crises, and celebrate each other's successes. This type of relationship becomes a safe base from which both can face the world, knowing they always have someone by their side who supports them.

Sign of Mutual Support: In a healthy relationship, you know your partner is there for you in times of need and that they will do their best to help you overcome difficulties. Likewise, you are ready to support the other, knowing that you are in this journey of life together.

Conclusion: The Beauty of a Healthy and Fulfilling Relationship

Recognizing a healthy and fulfilling relationship means being able to read the signs of balance, reciprocity, and care that make a bond truly special. It is a relationship that doesn't seek to change or control but values the other for who they are, offering a space of safety and mutual growth. It is a place where trust, respect, and open communication form the foundation of love that nurtures and enriches each day.

In a healthy relationship, we can fully be ourselves, free to grow and blossom together, knowing that, no matter what happens, we are loved and respected exactly for who we are.

Differences Between Romantic Love and Dependent Love

At first glance, romantic love and dependent love may seem like two sides of the same coin: both arise from the desire for connection, affection toward the other, and the will to create a deep bond. However, their roots lie in very different soils, and the results—a healthy relationship or a suffocating one—reflect their true nature. Understanding the difference between these two forms of love means learning to distinguish between a feeling that enriches and one that depletes, between a connection that liberates and one that traps.

1. Romantic Love: A Meeting Between Two Free Souls

Romantic love is a meeting place for two souls, where they recognize, choose, and enrich each other. It is a feeling born not from necessity or need but from the desire to share life with someone we love and respect. In romantic love, each partner is complete in themselves but chooses to walk alongside the other for the joy of sharing a journey, growing together while maintaining their individuality.

In a healthy romantic relationship, partners support each other without stifling the other's freedom. The bond is not a cage but a garden where both can flourish, nourished by mutual respect and the ability to grow as individuals. Romantic love is based on reciprocity: a natural flow of giving and receiving without pressure or stifling expectations. It creates a space of trust and safety where each can be themselves without fear of judgment or abandonment.

Romantic love celebrates differences, embraces vulnerabilities, and offers support in times of need without asking for anything in return. It's not about filling an inner void with the other person, but about sharing one's fullness with them. This kind of love imposes no conditions; it thrives on freedom, respect, and trust. Partners do not try to change each other but embrace the other's authenticity, allowing love to become a space for mutual expression and growth.

Sign of Romantic Love: In a romantic relationship, you feel free to be yourself and express your needs without fear of being judged or rejected. There is deep respect for your individuality, and your partner encourages you to grow and pursue your dreams without trying to control or limit you.

2. Dependent Love: A Bond of Need and Fear

Dependent love, on the other hand, does not stem from freedom but from fear. It is a feeling rooted in insecurity, the terror of being alone, and the belief that one is not enough without the other. While romantic love is an encounter between two people who choose each other in their autonomy, dependent love is a bond in which one or both partners cling to the other to fill an inner void. The other person becomes not a companion but a lifeline, something that cannot be done without in order to feel complete or secure.

In a dependent relationship, love is confused with the obsessive need for attention, validation, and constant presence. The boundaries between the two partners blur, and one or both begin to lose their identity. Dependent love becomes an emotional prison where the other is no longer someone with whom to share life but a crutch to lean on to avoid falling. The fear of abandonment is so strong that every gesture, every word of the other is monitored, interpreted, and often misunderstood.

Dependent love knows no freedom. Every emotional or physical distance is met with anxiety, and any sign of the other's independence is perceived as a threat. One feels suffocated by the thought that the other might leave or choose to live without them, creating a cycle of control and possessiveness. Dependent love doesn't build—it consumes: it consumes energy, trust, and, ultimately, the relationship itself. Partners don't grow together but cling to each other, often sinking in a sea of jealousy, insecurities, and emotional dependence.

Sign of Dependent Love: In a dependent relationship, you feel a constant need for validation, presence, and attention. You worry that the other might leave you or not love you enough, and this fear leads you to want to control their time, feelings, and choices. Your emotional well-being depends almost entirely on the other person's behavior.

3. Freedom vs. Possessiveness: A Fundamental Contrast

One of the key elements distinguishing romantic love from dependent love is the concept of freedom. In romantic love, each partner is free to be themselves, pursue their interests, and cultivate their individuality. Freedom is not seen as a threat but as a natural and essential element for the growth of the bond. Loving someone doesn't mean possessing them but accompanying them on their journey, allowing them to be fully themselves.

In dependent love, on the contrary, possessiveness takes over. The other's freedom is perceived as a danger, a potential source of abandonment or betrayal. One tries to control the other, needing to know where they are, who they are with, and what they are doing because any act of independence is feared as a precursor to the relationship's end. Possessiveness stems from fear and insecurity, eventually suffocating the partner and creating a spiral of jealousy, suspicion, and tension.

Sign of Freedom in Romantic Love: In a romantic relationship, you feel secure in your individuality, knowing that your partner respects your freedom to grow, change, and explore the world without feeling threatened or limited. You don't need to know every detail of their life to feel loved.

Sign of Possessiveness in Dependent Love: In a dependent relationship, you feel the need to control every aspect of your partner's life. Their independence frightens you, and you worry that if you're not always present, they might leave or find someone else.

4. The Balance Between Giving and Receiving

In romantic love, there is a natural balance between giving and receiving. Partners care for each other spontaneously, without expecting anything in return, knowing that love flows reciprocally. Love is not a game of trades or debts to settle—both give their best, not because they feel obligated, but because they derive joy from seeing the other happy. There is a genuine generosity that nourishes the relationship, creating a bond that enriches both partners.

In dependent love, on the other hand, giving and receiving are often unbalanced. One partner may feel compelled to sacrifice their own needs to maintain the relationship, while the other may demand constant attention and validation. This creates a toxic dynamic where sacrifice becomes the currency for obtaining love. In dependent love, there is often a sense of emotional exhaustion, as one or both partners feel they are not receiving what they need but don't know how to break free from the cycle of deprivation.

Sign of Balance in Romantic Love: In a romantic relationship, both partners feel fulfilled and respected. There is no sense of having to give too much or sacrificing oneself to maintain the bond because there is a natural flow of care and mutual attention.

Sign of Imbalance in Dependent Love: In a dependent relationship, one partner constantly feels like they must do more to keep the other, while the other demands more attention, affection, or validation without ever feeling truly satisfied.

Conclusion: Choosing the Love That Nourishes

The difference between romantic love and dependent love is subtle but crucial. Romantic love is an encounter between free souls who choose to walk together without giving up their individuality, while dependent love is a form of attachment born from fear and insecurity, trapping the partners in a suffocating dynamic.

Recognizing these differences allows us to make more conscious choices in our relationships, cultivating bonds that enrich and strengthen us rather than imprison us. In a world where love is often idealized or misunderstood, choosing to love freely, respectfully, and reciprocally is the first step toward building a healthy and fulfilling relationship, allowing both individuals and the couple to thrive.

Mature Relationships: Individual and Couple Growth

Mature relationships are like ancient oak trees, deeply rooted in trust, respect, and mutual understanding, yet flexible in their growth, reaching new heights of discovery and development. A mature relationship is not only measured by the time spent together but by the depth with which two people support each other on the journey of life, while also maintaining a sacred space for their individual growth. This delicate balance is essential: on one side, the intimacy and closeness of the couple; on the other, the respect for each partner's autonomy and personal evolution.

In a society often obsessed with quick and superficial relationships, the idea of a mature relationship stands out as a beacon of stability and wisdom. It goes beyond initial passion or classic romantic dynamics, reaching a dimension of awareness, collaboration, and mutual growth, where both partners not only support but enrich each other.

1. The Balance Between Intimacy and Freedom: The Heart of the Relationship

The first distinguishing feature of a mature relationship is the ability to balance intimacy with individual freedom. In an immature relationship, there is often fear of losing the other, or a tendency to live solely for the partner, stifling one's desires, needs, or personal ambitions. However, in a mature relationship, intimacy is never a threat to freedom. Instead, the couple learns to cultivate a space where each partner is encouraged to grow individually, while the connection between them remains strong and stable.

In a mature relationship, each partner is free to explore their passions, pursue their dreams, and grow as an individual, knowing that this won't weaken the bond, but strengthen it. Personal freedom is not seen as a threat, but as an essential component to keeping the relationship alive and dynamic. The more each partner feels fulfilled in their individual life, the more the relationship becomes fertile ground for companionship and shared experiences.

This balance is built on deep mutual trust, born from the awareness that the relationship does not depend on control or possession, but on respect and the conscious choice to grow together. Every moment spent together is precious because both know they have chosen to be there, not out of obligation, but out of the authentic desire to share.

Sign of Balance: In a mature relationship, you don't feel the need to control or limit your partner. Each has their own space to grow and explore, and this is seen as enriching the couple, not as a threat.

2. Individual Growth as a Pillar of the Relationship

In a mature relationship, individual growth is not sacrificed to maintain the bond. Instead, it is recognized as an indispensable element for the relationship's longevity and vitality. When each partner commits to cultivating their identity and personal well-being, the relationship becomes a space of mutual enrichment, where both can bring the best version of themselves.

Individual growth can manifest in many ways: professional achievement, the development of new passions or interests, or personal evolution such as mindfulness practices, improving self-esteem, or emotional healing. What makes a relationship mature is the ability to support this growth without competition or envy. A partner's success is not seen as a threat but as a source of inspiration and pride for the other.

Individual growth is the lifeblood that keeps the relationship alive, as it allows each partner to bring new energy and perspectives into the relationship. When both people are committed to bettering themselves, the relationship becomes dynamic, with constant curiosity and discovery.

Sign of Individual Growth: In a mature relationship, you feel your partner encourages you to grow, develop new skills, and pursue your dreams. There's never the feeling of having to choose between personal evolution and the relationship because you know both can coexist.

3. Conscious Communication: The Dialogue That Nourishes

Another hallmark of a mature relationship is conscious communication. While immature relationships are often characterized by misunderstandings, silences, manipulations, or emotional clashes, in a mature relationship, dialogue is open, honest, and respectful. There's no fear in expressing feelings, doubts, or vulnerabilities, because both partners know the other will listen without judgment.

Conscious communication is not just about telling the truth but how the truth is conveyed. In a mature relationship, partners are mindful of the words they use, knowing that dialogue is a tool not only for resolving conflicts but for creating connection and intimacy. Conversations go beyond the practical aspects of daily life and become a space where both can share their dreams, fears, and deepest aspirations.

In a mature relationship, there's no fear of conflict. In fact, conflicts are seen as an opportunity to grow together. Both partners know that a disagreement is not a threat to the bond but a chance to better understand each other and strengthen the relationship. Conscious communication allows challenges to be faced with maturity, without resorting to power plays or emotional manipulation.

Sign of Conscious Communication: In a mature relationship, you feel heard and understood when you speak. You know you can express your feelings without fear of being misunderstood or ignored, and you are willing to listen to your partner with the same attention and respect.

4. Mutual Support: A Life Partnership

A mature relationship is a true partnership, an alliance in life. In it, partners support each other through difficult times as well as moments of joy. They're not just present for the easy moments but offer their support when it's needed most, creating a safe space where both can count on one another.

Mutual support is not just emotional but extends into daily life, dreams, and ambitions. In a mature relationship, there is a commitment to lift each other up, to help each partner achieve their goals and overcome difficulties. There's no sense of competition, only the awareness that one's success is a success for both.

This dynamic of mutual support creates a foundation of security and trust, where both partners know they can rely on each other. There's no doubt about each other's dedication and commitment because the relationship is built on a mutual agreement of support and care that is renewed daily.

Sign of Mutual Support: In a mature relationship, you feel that your partner is your biggest supporter. In difficult times, you don't feel alone because you know the other will be by your side, ready to give you strength and encouragement.

5. The Constant Evolution of the Couple: Growing Together

A mature relationship is never static. It doesn't settle for staying the same over time but is in constant evolution. As each partner grows and transforms individually, the couple also grows and renews itself. A mature relationship is like a flowing river: it doesn't fear change but embraces it, knowing that it is a natural part of the journey.

Growing together doesn't mean always doing everything together or sharing every single aspect of life. It means being there for each other, even when personal paths seem to diverge temporarily. Growing together is an act of trust: knowing that despite changes, the bond remains strong because it's built on solid foundations of love, respect, and mutual support.

In a mature relationship, both partners learn to celebrate not only moments of joy but also moments of transformation. Every challenge overcome together becomes a milestone, a symbol of the couple's strength and resilience.

Sign of Couple Growth: In a mature relationship, you feel that the couple evolves together. Difficult times don't weaken the bond but make it stronger, and change is seen as an opportunity to know each other better and grow together.

Conclusion: The Beauty of Mature Relationships

Mature relationships are a refuge of love, companionship, and mutual growth. They are not immune to difficulties but have the capacity to transform each challenge into an opportunity for evolution and strengthening the bond. The beauty of a mature relationship lies in its flexibility and depth: it's a place where each partner can fully be themselves, grow as an individual, and, at the same time, create a rich and fulfilling life together.

In a mature relationship, individual growth and couple growth are not in conflict but feed each other, creating a bond that not only withstands the test of time but flourishes with it, becoming ever stronger, more authentic, and more radiant.

Learning to Live Love in a Free and Authentic Way

Living love in a free and authentic way is one of the most powerful and transformative experiences we can have. It is a journey that leads us to overcome the illusions and fears that often envelop our relationships, allowing us to embrace a love that is not based on possession, dependence, or expectations, but on the full expression of oneself and the other. Authentic love is like a river flowing without obstacles: it is fluid, nourishing, and finds its strength in its freedom.

Learning to live love this way means leaving behind old dynamics of control and insecurity, stepping into a space of acceptance where each person can be themselves, loved for who they are—without masks, without fear. In this kind of love, there is room for vulnerability, growth, and transformation, and each encounter becomes an opportunity for mutual discovery, a shared path toward greater awareness and fulfillment.

1. Authenticity: Being Yourself Without Masks

Authenticity is the foundation of free love. Being authentic means showing yourself as you truly are, without trying to hide your vulnerabilities or build an idealized version of yourself to please the other. Authentic love doesn't arise from the perfect image we wish to project, but from the truth of who we are. When two people love each other authentically, they have the courage to reveal themselves, to share their fears, uncertainties, and dreams, knowing they will be embraced without judgment.

Being authentic in love requires vulnerability, and this vulnerability is what makes love so deep and true. We often fear showing who we really are because we're afraid of not being accepted or being seen as not enough. But in authentic love, there is a deep understanding that the other is not seeking perfection but truth. This truth, with all its imperfections, is what allows the bond to become truly intimate and liberating.

Sign of Authenticity in Love: In an authentic relationship, you don't feel the need to hide who you are. You can freely express your thoughts, emotions, and desires, knowing that the other loves and accepts you for your true essence. There are no power plays or manipulation attempts, just the sincerity of two souls meeting and respecting each other.

2. Free Love: Letting Go of Control and Possessiveness

Free love is love that doesn't cling, that doesn't seek to possess or control the other. Often, when we love, we fear losing the other, and this fear leads us to try to control the relationship, the time, the spaces, and the emotions. But free love is based on trust and the awareness that love cannot be held or forced. It's like the wind: the more we try to grasp it, the more it slips away, but if we let it flow, it surrounds us with all its sweetness.

In a relationship based on freedom, the other is not property but a companion on the journey. Both partners are free to be themselves, to cultivate their interests, and to live their lives with authenticity. Freedom in love does not mean living separately or distantly but recognizing that each person has the right to follow their own path without fear of judgment or limitation. This type of freedom enriches the relationship because it allows the couple to grow together while maintaining the integrity of their individuality.

Possessiveness, on the other hand, suffocates love. When we try to control the other, when we fear they will slip away or distance themselves, we are denying their freedom—and ultimately, our own. Free love teaches us to let go of these dynamics, to trust the bond we've created, and to recognize that love flourishes only in a space of autonomy and reciprocity.

Sign of Free Love: In free love, you don't feel the need to control the other or know every detail of their life. You trust the bond you've created and respect your partner's freedom to be themselves, without constraints or impositions.

3. Unconditional Love: Loving Without Expectations

One of the greatest challenges in love is learning to love without conditions. Often, even unconsciously, we place expectations on the other: we want them to behave in a certain way, to fulfill our needs, or to respond to our demands for attention and affection. However, authentic love is love that asks for nothing in return. It is love that is offered generously, given without expecting anything back, knowing that the joy of loving lies in the act itself, not in what we receive.

Loving unconditionally means recognizing the other's wholeness, accepting even what we cannot change or control. In this kind of love, we don't seek to alter the other or mold them into what we desire but embrace them for who they are, with all their imperfections and uniqueness. It's a love that is not based on unrealistic expectations but on the understanding that the other is a person separate from us, with their own desires, dreams, and needs.

When we love unconditionally, our love becomes independent of the other's behavior or what we receive in return. This doesn't mean tolerating everything but recognizing that love is not a transaction—it is a free and spontaneous gift that is renewed each day by the conscious choice to love.

Sign of Unconditional Love: In an unconditional relationship, you don't expect the other to conform to an ideal or fulfill every need. You embrace them for who they are, and your love doesn't depend on how they act or what they give in return. You love generously, accepting that love is a free exchange, not a demand.

4. Vulnerability: The Courage to Be Fragile Together

Authentic love requires vulnerability. We often think that loving means being strong, having everything under control, but the deepest love arises when we allow ourselves to be fragile in front of each other. In an authentic relationship, you feel safe sharing your fears, uncertainties, and flaws. There is no need to hide the most delicate parts of yourself because you know the other will welcome you with kindness and understanding.

Being vulnerable means opening your heart, lowering your defenses, allowing the other to see who you truly are. This can be frightening because vulnerability exposes us to the risk of being hurt. But it is in vulnerability that love finds its true strength. When we allow ourselves to be vulnerable, we create a deeper, more intimate bond, where there are no barriers between us and the other. Authentic love is a place where we can be imperfect, and that's okay, because we know the other loves us for our humanity.

Vulnerability is not weakness but courage. It is the courage to say, "This is who I am, with all my fears and insecurities. Will you accept me?" And when the other responds with a yes, love becomes a place of healing and profound connection.

Sign of Vulnerability in Love: In an authentic relationship, you feel free to share your fears and insecurities without fear of judgment or rejection. You know the other will embrace your fragility with care and respect, creating a space of deep intimacy.

5. Reciprocity: A Meeting of Souls That Support Each Other

Living love in a free and authentic way also means understanding the value of reciprocity. Love cannot exist in one direction: it must be an exchange, a continuous flow of giving and receiving, care and support. In authentic love, both partners are committed to nurturing the bond, caring for the other with the same attention with which they care for themselves. There is no partner who always gives and one who always receives—both actively contribute to the well-being of the relationship.

Reciprocity is not about quantity but intention. It means being present for the other in times of need, but also knowing when it's time to receive without feeling guilty. It's an exchange of energy where love flows freely in both directions, creating a balance that enriches both partners.

Sign of Reciprocity in Love: In an authentic relationship, you feel the other is there for you just as much as you are for them. There is a natural balance in giving and receiving, and both are committed to nurturing the bond with love, attention, and care.

Conclusion: The Art of Living Free and Authentic Love

Learning to live love in a free and authentic way is a journey toward a deeper connection with ourselves and with others. It is a path that requires awareness, trust, and courage, but it leads us to experience love that goes beyond conventions, fears, and expectations. It is love that allows us to be fully present, to live each moment with authenticity, to embrace the other in their wholeness, and to love without limits or conditions.

In this kind of love, we find the freedom to be who we truly are—without masks or compromises—and the joy of sharing our lives with someone who sees us, accepts us, and loves us for who we are. It is love that doesn't hold back but liberates, that doesn't demand but offers, and, for this reason, becomes one of the richest and most fulfilling experiences we can live.

art 5: Living Love in a Healthy and Autonomous WayChapter 15

The Future of Your Emotional Life

How to Maintain Emotional Balance Over Time

Maintaining emotional balance over time is like navigating a constantly changing sea. Some days, the waters are calm and clear, allowing us to move forward with ease, while at other times, the waves rise menacingly, testing our inner stability. However, just as an experienced sailor knows how to stay the course during storms, each of us can learn to find our emotional center, that place of inner peace and strength that allows us to face life's challenges without being overwhelmed by them.

Emotional balance is not a fixed state but a constant movement of adaptation and awareness. It is the art of recognizing our emotions, accepting them without judgment, and learning to respond to situations with calmness and clarity, even when everything around us seems turbulent. It is a delicate dance between the external world, which often tests us, and the internal world, where we can find our refuge, our strength, and our safe space.

1. Self-Awareness: Listening to Your Emotions

The first step to maintaining emotional balance is developing a deep sense of self-awareness. Often, we get so caught up in the fast pace of daily life that we end up ignoring what is happening inside us. However, to find balance, it is essential to learn to listen to our emotions, recognize them, and understand their origins. Emotions are not enemies to be fought but messengers that speak to us about our needs, fears, and insecurities.

Being aware of what we feel means pausing, taking a deep breath, and asking, "What am I feeling right now?" Awareness allows us to connect with our emotions without being overwhelmed by them. Instead of reacting impulsively to situations, we learn to recognize what is happening within and can respond with more clarity and calmness.

This ability to observe ourselves prevents emotional highs and lows, helping us avoid being swept away by the moment. It's not about repressing or denying emotions but accepting and understanding them, letting them flow without being drowned by them.

Emotional Awareness Exercise: Each day, take a few minutes to pause and ask yourself what you are feeling in that moment. Don't judge the emotions that arise—observe them with curiosity and acceptance. This practice will help you develop greater awareness of your emotional states and recognize them before they become overwhelming.

2. The Art of Emotional Detachment: Responding, Not Reacting

Emotional detachment doesn't mean indifference or coldness; rather, it's the ability not to be swept away by emotions when they become particularly intense. Often, when we face a difficult or stressful situation, we react impulsively, letting anger, fear, or frustration take control. However, maintaining emotional balance requires us to develop the skill of responding to situations rather than reacting automatically.

Responding means taking a pause, observing the emotion as it arises, and then choosing how to act. Instead of being swept away by emotion like a raging river, we find a detached perspective that allows us to see things more clearly. This detachment helps us stay calm, even in challenging situations, giving us space to reflect and act consciously.

Emotional detachment is a form of self-control, but it's not repression. We acknowledge the emotion, accept it, but choose not to be dominated by it. This ability to create a small gap between emotion and reaction is what allows us to maintain balance, even under pressure.

Emotional Detachment Exercise: When you feel overwhelmed by a strong emotion, pause for a few seconds. Take three deep breaths and imagine mentally distancing yourself from the situation, as if you were observing it from the outside. This will give you the time needed to respond with calmness and awareness.

3. The Power of Breath: Staying Grounded in the Body

Breathing is one of the most powerful tools for maintaining emotional balance. Often, when faced with emotional stress, we tend to breathe shallowly or even hold our breath. However, breath is the key to staying grounded in the present and calming the nervous system.

Learning to breathe deeply and mindfully helps release tension and return to a state of calm and stability. Conscious breathing reconnects us to our body, allowing us to feel present and grounded in the here and now, instead of being swept away by anxious thoughts or worries about the past or future.

When we practice deep breathing, we send a message to our body that we are safe, that there is no need to engage in a fight-or-flight response. This helps reduce anxiety, fear, and emotional tension, allowing us to stay calm even in moments of difficulty.

Conscious Breathing Exercise: Whenever you feel stressed or overwhelmed by emotions, stop and take five deep breaths. Inhale slowly through your nose, expanding your diaphragm, and then exhale completely through your mouth. Focus on the movement of the breath and the sensation of relaxation it brings.

4. Self-Care: Creating Rituals for Well-Being

Maintaining emotional balance also requires taking care of your mental and physical well-being. Emotions are closely linked to the body, and when we neglect our physical self, our emotional state suffers. Creating self-care rituals is essential to maintaining a state of balance over time.

This can include a variety of practices, from regular physical activity, which helps release accumulated tension, to meditation, which calms the mind and reduces stress. Taking time to cultivate personal hobbies and passions or simply enjoying moments of pleasure and relaxation is crucial for maintaining emotional stability.

Self-care is a way to recharge your energy and create a space of calm and serenity in daily life. When we take care of ourselves, we are offering love and respect to ourselves, which directly reflects on our ability to manage emotions in a healthy and balanced way.

Self-Care Exercise: Dedicate at least 20 minutes each day to a personal care practice. This could be a walk, a yoga session, reading a book, or a relaxing bath. These small moments of daily care will help you maintain a constant level of emotional well-being.

5. Gratitude and Forgiveness: Healing the Past to Live in the Present

To maintain emotional balance over time, it's crucial to learn to let go of the weight of the past. Often, the emotions that destabilize us are rooted in old wounds, resentments, or regrets that we haven't yet addressed. Practicing gratitude and forgiveness helps us heal these wounds and find peace.

Gratitude teaches us to shift our focus from problems or difficulties to the positives in our lives. When we focus on what we are grateful for, we change our emotional perspective and find greater inner stability. Forgiveness, on the other hand, allows us to let go of the past, freeing ourselves from the burden of negative emotions and opening up to a new emotional lightness.

Learning to forgive doesn't mean justifying what happened, but freeing ourselves from the attachment to the pain that event caused. It is an act of inner liberation that allows us to fully return to the present, without being tied to what we can no longer change.

Gratitude and Forgiveness Exercise: Each evening, before going to sleep, take a moment to reflect on three things you are grateful for. Then, think of a situation or person you want to forgive, even just a little. Mentally say the words, "I choose to forgive," and release the emotional weight attached to that memory.

6. Resilience: Embracing Change with Flexibility

Emotional balance doesn't mean avoiding difficulties or living without challenges but learning to face them with resilience. Life is constantly changing, and maintaining emotional balance requires the ability to adapt with flexibility. Resilience allows us to view moments of crisis not as defeats but as opportunities for personal growth and evolution.

Being resilient means accepting that difficult emotions are part of life and learning to manage them without running from them. It means finding the courage to face hard times with an open heart, knowing that every storm passes and that, in the end, we can emerge stronger and more self-aware.

Resilience Exercise: Whenever you face a challenge, try asking yourself, "What can I learn from this situation? How can I grow through this experience?" This change in perspective will help you see crises as part of your growth journey.

Conclusion: The Journey Toward Emotional Balance

Maintaining emotional balance over time is a journey that requires awareness, self-care, and a constant ability to adapt. It is an inner journey that leads us to better understand our emotions, learn to manage them wisely, and find within ourselves that quiet strength that allows us to face life with serenity and compassion. When we learn to live with emotional balance, we discover a new inner freedom, a peace that allows us to navigate life's storms with an open heart and a clear mind, knowing that no matter what happens, we can always return to our center.

Part 5: Living Love in a Healthy and Autonomous WayChapter 15

The Future of Your Emotional Life

Continuing the Journey of Personal Growth: Life as Constant Evolution

Life is an endless journey, a ceaseless dance between who we are and who we are becoming. With each step, we leave behind old versions of ourselves and open ourselves to change, transformation, and the discovery of new aspects of our being. Continuing the path of personal growth means accepting life as a constant evolution, where there is no definitive destination, but only stages marking our journey, each with its own set of experiences, lessons, and awareness.

Personal growth is an inner journey that takes us deep into our being, where we can recognize our vulnerabilities, enhance our strengths, and become more aware and complete each day. It is a path that requires courage, as it often invites us to look inside ourselves with honesty, confront our fears and limitations, and choose to change what no longer serves us. But it is also a path that leads to greater freedom and fulfillment because it allows us to live more authentically, more consciously, and more in alignment with our true desires.

1. Acceptance of Change: Embracing Uncertainty and Transformation

One of the fundamental aspects of personal growth is the acceptance of change. Life is in constant evolution: people, situations, emotions, and even our dreams change over time. However, we often cling to the past, to certainties, to what we know, because change frightens us. Yet, it is precisely uncertainty that offers us the opportunity to grow.

Every change, even those that may seem painful or difficult at first, brings with it a new perspective, a new possibility to evolve. Embracing change means being willing to let go of what no longer serves us, to make room for new experiences, and to trust in the flow of life. When we learn to accept that change is a natural and inevitable part of our existence, we free ourselves from the fear of losing control and discover the beauty of renewal.

Every phase of life offers us new challenges and opportunities for growth. Nothing remains static, and this is the gift of personal evolution: every day is a new beginning, every experience is a chance to become a more conscious and true version of ourselves.

Exercise for Embracing Change: Whenever you find yourself facing a significant life transition, whether it be a change in relationships, work, or beliefs, ask yourself, "What can I learn from this situation? How can I use this change to evolve?" This will help you see change as an opportunity rather than a threat.

2. Awareness as an Inner Compass: Living in the Here and Now

Awareness is the key to progressing on the path of personal growth. Living in a state of presence allows us to recognize our emotions, thoughts, and reactions and make decisions that are more aligned with our inner truth. Growth cannot happen without awareness, as it is only through self-observation that we can identify what needs to be changed and improved.

Life constantly offers us lessons and opportunities to grow, but to seize them, we must be present in the moment. Awareness invites us not to dwell in the past, where regrets and old wounds remain, nor to project ourselves into the future, where anxieties and uncertainties dominate, but to live fully in the here and now. This present moment is the only ground on which we can build our evolution, the only space where we can act, decide, and choose who we want to become.

When we are self-aware, we can observe without judgment our limiting thoughts, fears, and destructive habits and gradually transform them in a positive way. Awareness thus becomes a compass that guides us along the path of growth, helping us make more authentic choices and live a life more aligned with our values.

Awareness Exercise: Each day, dedicate a few minutes to practicing awareness. Sit in silence, focus on your breath, and observe the thoughts and emotions that arise without judging them. This will help you develop a stronger connection with the present moment and make more conscious decisions.

3. The Strength of Vulnerability: Embracing Your Fragility to Grow

Often, in our culture, personal growth is associated with strength and the ability to overcome obstacles. However, one of the deepest dimensions of growth is the ability to be vulnerable. Vulnerability is not weakness, but an act of courage that allows us to accept our fragilities, to recognize that we are not perfect, and that this is okay. It is only through vulnerability that we can create a space for healing, both for ourselves and for our relationships.

When we learn to embrace our vulnerability, we stop hiding the parts of ourselves that we consider imperfect or flawed. We are finally free to be authentic and live with greater lightness. Personal growth does not only happen by overcoming difficulties but also by recognizing and accepting our emotions without repressing or ignoring them.

Being vulnerable makes us more human, more connected to others, and to our true essence. Vulnerability opens us to the possibility of learning, improving, and growing because it allows us to look inside ourselves without judgment but with compassion and self-acceptance.

Vulnerability Exercise: Whenever you feel fragile or vulnerable, try not to hide these emotions but express them honestly, at least to yourself. Write in a journal about what you are feeling without censoring or judging your emotions. This will help you develop greater self-acceptance.

4. The Power of Resilience: Turning Adversity into Opportunity

Resilience is one of the most valuable qualities we can develop on our personal growth journey. Life, with its challenges and difficulties, often presents us with moments of crisis that may seem insurmountable. But it is precisely in these moments that we have the opportunity to grow and discover a new strength within ourselves. Resilience is the ability to bounce back from adversity, to turn pain into wisdom, and to see failures not as defeats but as lessons that make us stronger.

Being resilient doesn't mean not suffering or avoiding difficulties. It means finding within ourselves the resources to adapt, overcome challenges, and evolve through them. Resilience allows us to view every experience, even the most painful ones, as an opportunity to learn something new about ourselves and life.

When we face a challenge, we can choose to remain stuck in the pain or use it as a springboard for change. Resilience teaches us not to fear the dark moments but to recognize them as an integral part of our growth journey.

Resilience Exercise: When facing a challenge or difficulty, ask yourself, "How can I turn this experience into an opportunity for growth? What can I learn from this situation?" This will help you develop a resilient mindset and see difficulties as steps in your evolutionary journey.

5. Self-Love: The Foundation of Growth

Self-love is the fertile ground from which all personal growth flourishes. Without love and respect for ourselves, every attempt at improvement risks being superficial or driven by the anxiety of conforming to external standards. Self-love is the foundation upon which to build an authentic life, as it allows us to accept ourselves as we are, with our strengths and weaknesses, and work to improve, not to please others but to live in harmony with our true essence.

Loving oneself doesn't mean being indulgent or selfish but taking care of one's emotional, physical, and spiritual well-being. It means recognizing that we are worthy of love and respect, regardless of our mistakes or failures. When we develop deep self-love, we stop seeking external validation and find within ourselves the strength and courage to evolve authentically.

Self-love allows us to make choices more aligned with our true desires, set healthy boundaries in relationships, and create a personal growth space where we can thrive without fear.

Self-Love Exercise: Each day, take a moment to practice self-compassion. Look at yourself in the mirror and speak words of encouragement and love to yourself. Remind yourself that you are worthy of love, no matter what you've done or how you feel. This simple gesture will help you cultivate deep and sincere love for yourself.

6. Life as a Journey: There Is No Final Destination

Finally, to continue the path of personal growth, it's important to remember that life is a journey, not a destination. We often set goals to reach as if growth were a fixed point to conquer. But the truth is that growth is a continuous process, without end. Every time we reach a new level of awareness or achievement, we realize that there is still more to explore, more to learn.

This doesn't mean we can't feel satisfied or complete. On the contrary, it means we can live with the awareness that life offers us infinite opportunities to evolve, discover new parts of ourselves, and expand our view of the world. Personal growth isn't an obligation but a conscious choice to continue discovering, learning, and transforming.

Exercise for Living Life as a Journey: Each month, take a moment to reflect on what you've learned in recent weeks and how you've grown. Celebrate your progress and open yourself to the possibility that there is always something new to discover and learn.

Conclusion: The Infinite Journey of Personal Growth

Continuing the path of personal growth means living life as a process of constant evolution. It is a journey that invites us to discover more and more about who we are, to embrace change, and to find strength in vulnerability. Life is not a series of goals to be achieved but a continuous flow of experiences that transform us, enrich us, and lead us toward greater awareness and fulfillment.

In this journey, there is no final destination, only the beauty of the path itself. Each day offers the opportunity to grow, learn, and evolve, and it is up to us to embrace this opportunity with an open heart and a mind ready to explore new horizons. Life, in all its complexity, is the greatest teacher we can have, and personal growth is its most precious lesson.

Chapter 16: The Freedom to Love Without Depending

Loving without depending is like dancing in a vast, open space where each step is moved by freedom and not by fear, by the desire to share and not by the need to be completed. It's a love that doesn't cling, doesn't constantly seek validation, but finds its strength in the inner fullness of the one who loves. Loving in this way is an act of mutual liberation, a celebration of the choice to be together, not because the other person saves or defines us, but because with them we can truly be ourselves.

Emotional dependence, on the other hand, is like an invisible chain that binds us to the other out of fear of loneliness, emptiness, or not feeling good enough. It makes us feel incomplete, as if only through the other can we find our worth. But authentic love, the one born from freedom, invites us to be whole in ourselves in order to share that completeness with the other, without trying to possess, control, or make them a refuge from our insecurities.

1. Love as a Conscious Choice

Loving without depending means first of all choosing to love consciously, not out of need. In a relationship based on dependence, love often arises from the fear of being alone, from seeking in the other a sort of compensation for our own shortcomings or fears. This type of love is fragile because it rests on unstable foundations, on a continuous search for reassurance that the other can never fully provide.

Free love, on the other hand, is an act of will. We choose to love because the other enriches our life, not because they fill it. In this freedom of choice, there is no fear of loss but the joy of sharing. We don't love to heal our wounds but to celebrate the personal and mutual growth together. Each day, the decision to stay together is renewed, not out of need or dependency, but because that love is a space for growth, support, and mutual respect.

- **Sign of conscious love**: In a free relationship, every gesture of affection, every kind word, every shared moment is a choice, not a duty. There is no pressure or sense of sacrifice, only the desire to be together for the joy of it, because the other represents a precious part of your life, without being the absolute center.

2. The Freedom to Be Yourself

Another distinctive sign of free love is the ability to be fully yourself, without fear of losing the other. When we love without depending, we don't feel the need to adapt or hide parts of ourselves out of fear of not being enough or being abandoned. Instead, we feel free to show our vulnerabilities, dreams, and even our flaws, knowing that the other accepts us for who we are without wanting to change us.

In love based on dependence, on the other hand, we often end up conforming to an ideal image to meet the other's expectations. We fear that if we're not perfect or don't meet their desires, we may be rejected. This creates an invisible cage where we hide behind a mask to avoid vulnerability, to avoid the risk of rejection. But authentic love doesn't require perfection, it requires authenticity.

Free love is a safe space where each person can be vulnerable without fear, where flaws and imperfections are not a reason for separation but an opportunity for deeper connection. In this kind of love, we love each other for who we are, not for who we should be.

- **Sign of inner freedom**: In a relationship based on free love, you feel comfortable expressing your true feelings and thoughts. You don't feel the need to hide who you are or change to be loved. You know the other appreciates you in your entirety, and this gives you the freedom to fully be yourself.

3. Love That Doesn't Hold but Liberates

Free love does not try to hold onto the other, to control them, or to possess them. On the contrary, it leaves room for individual growth and evolution. Emotional dependence, however, is marked by the fear of loss, by the constant need for presence and reassurance. We fear that if the other is too free, they may drift away or abandon us, creating a vicious cycle of control, jealousy, and possessiveness.

But authentic love is a force that liberates. When we love without depending, we realize that love cannot be forced or held back. What restrains suffocates, but what frees allows to flourish. In a free relationship, we give the other the space to pursue their interests, to cultivate their individuality, knowing that love doesn't diminish with distance but strengthens in mutual trust.

This doesn't mean that free love doesn't have moments of difficulty or fear, but the difference lies in the ability to face these challenges without imposing limits on the other. We address our fears with dialogue, with understanding, but without trying to restrict the other or force them to behave a certain way to meet our needs. Free love lets the other be, and in that freedom, a deep trust is built.

- **Sign of love that liberates**: In free love, you feel at peace letting the other have their own spaces, interests, and moments of independence. You don't feel the need to control them or to always be present because you know that love doesn't depend on the amount of time spent together but on the quality of connection and mutual trust.

4. Personal Growth as the Foundation of Love

One of the most beautiful aspects of loving without depending is the possibility of growing together without losing your individuality. When we are in a dependent relationship, personal growth is often set aside, sacrificed in the name of the relationship. We end up giving up our dreams, our desires because we fear the other won't approve or that by dedicating ourselves to ourselves, we might jeopardize the stability of the relationship.

But in free love, each partner is encouraged to follow their own path of personal growth. Love is not a cage that imprisons but a garden where each person can cultivate their talents, passions, and desires, knowing the other will be there to support, not limit. This kind of love is based on the understanding that the true strength of the bond lies in the ability to support each other, even in moments of individual change or growth.

When both partners grow and evolve, love enriches itself because a deep connection is created that isn't based on immobility or stagnation but on continuous evolution. Loving without depending means celebrating the other's individuality, knowing that personal growth is not a threat to the relationship but an enrichment.

- **Sign of mutual growth**: In a free relationship, you feel encouraged to pursue your dreams and ambitions. You know the other supports you on your growth journey and you don't feel you have to sacrifice yourself to maintain the relationship. At the same time, you support the other in their personal evolution, creating a space of mutual inspiration.

5. Vulnerability and the Strength of Free Love

Loving without depending also requires the courage to be vulnerable. Often, we think that freedom in love implies detachment or coldness, but in reality, it's the opposite: free love is full because it's based on trust and the ability to reveal oneself as we are without fear of losing the other. True freedom arises from shared vulnerability, from the ability to open up to the other without masks or barriers, knowing that even in difficulties, we can support each other without stifling one another.

Vulnerability in free love is what allows for a deep and authentic connection. When we are not bound by emotional dependence, we can explore our feelings with greater transparency and authenticity, knowing that love is not conditioned by our being perfect or strong but by our ability to be present and real. In this vulnerability, we find a strength that allows us to love with an open heart, without fear of being judged or abandoned.

- **Sign of shared vulnerability**: In a relationship based on free love, you feel comfortable showing your deepest emotions without fear of rejection. You know the other will accept you with understanding, and together you can face even the difficult moments, knowing the strength of the relationship lies in its authenticity.

Conclusion: The Art of Loving Without Depending

Loving without depending is an art, a journey toward a new awareness of self and the other. It's a love that nourishes itself on freedom, conscious choice, and mutual trust. In this space, love becomes a force that doesn't imprison but liberates, not because it demands something in return, but because it finds its richness in the sharing of two complete individuals who choose to walk together without needing to lean on one another to stay balanced.

The freedom to love without depending doesn't mean loving less or with less intensity but loving with greater awareness, with an open and vulnerable heart, ready to embrace the other in their entirety without needing to possess or change them. It's the kind of love that allows each person to flourish, despite or perhaps precisely because of the freedom given to the other, creating a space for growth, respect, and authentic connection.

The Importance of Staying Aware and Vigilant of Your Emotions

Emotions are like the wind: invisible, ever-changing, capable of sweeping us up with sudden force or brushing us gently like a breeze. They are constant companions, shaping our thoughts, actions, and perceptions of the world. Yet, we often let emotions carry us away without truly being aware of their presence and power. Learning to remain vigilant and aware of our emotions means becoming the captain of our own soul, able to navigate the inner seas without being overwhelmed by sudden waves of passion or impulse.

Being aware of your emotions doesn't mean suppressing or rigidly controlling them, but rather observing, recognizing, and embracing them with compassion and emotional intelligence. It is an act of profound inner maturity because it involves being present with oneself, listening to the silent language of the heart, and responding to this language with clarity, without being swept away by automatic or unconscious reactions. In this way, even the most intense and destabilizing emotions can be transformed into valuable guides for personal growth.

1. Emotions as an Inner Compass: Listening to the Heart's Messages

Emotions, often seen as unstable or uncontrollable forces, are actually an inner compass guiding us through life's complexities. Each emotion carries an important message, offering insight into what we are experiencing, what is affecting us, and how we are reacting to the outside world. For example, anger may signal that our boundaries have been crossed; sadness invites us to reflect on a loss or unmet need; joy points us toward our most authentic desires.

Being aware of our emotions means learning to decipher these messages, not running from them but pausing to listen. Often, we are tempted to ignore or suppress uncomfortable emotions like fear or pain, because we fear being overwhelmed by them. However, when we take the time to sit with our emotions and explore them with curiosity and kindness, we can gain a deeper understanding of ourselves and our most profound needs.

Emotions speak to us subtly, and if we are not attentive, we risk misunderstanding them or acting impulsively, without truly grasping what is happening inside. Emotional vigilance allows us to pause before reacting, to observe what we are feeling, and to ask ourselves, "What is this emotion trying to tell me?" Only then can we use emotions as a compass, rather than being unconsciously led by them.

- **Emotional listening exercise**: When you feel a strong emotion, pause for a few minutes and ask yourself, "What message is this emotion bringing me? What is it trying to tell me?" Take note of what arises and see how this awareness can help you respond more balancedly.

2. Emotional Vigilance: Avoiding Being Overwhelmed by Sudden Reactions

Remaining vigilant over your emotions means developing the ability to observe without immediately reacting. Often, when faced with a difficult or stressful situation, we react automatically, letting the emotion of the moment take control. However, when we learn to be aware of what we are feeling, we can create space between the emotion and our reaction, a space where we can choose how to act rather than responding impulsively.

Emotional vigilance is a form of conscious self-control—not in the sense of repressing emotions, but of managing them in a healthy, productive way. For example, when we feel anger, we may be tempted to react immediately with words or actions we might later regret. But if we remain vigilant, we can recognize the rising anger, take a moment to breathe and reflect, and then choose how to express that emotion in a way that doesn't harm ourselves or others.

This type of vigilance helps us avoid becoming slaves to our emotions. It allows us to stay centered, even in difficult situations, and to respond with maturity and compassion, both toward ourselves and others.

- **Emotional vigilance exercise**: When you feel a strong emotion like anger or fear, try taking three deep breaths before acting. Use that moment to observe the emotion, acknowledge it, and ask yourself how you want to respond, rather than reacting impulsively.

3. Awareness of the Emotional Cycle: Every Emotion Has a Beginning and an End

An important aspect of emotional awareness is understanding that every emotion has a natural cycle: it begins, grows, peaks, and then slowly fades away. When we are overwhelmed by a strong emotion, it may seem as though it will never end, that it will continue to dominate us forever. But the truth is that emotions, like waves, have a rhythm: if we learn not to resist and not to react immediately, we will find that the emotion itself will eventually start to subside.

Awareness of the emotional cycle allows us to face even the most difficult emotions with greater calm. Knowing that a feeling of anger, sadness, or fear will not last forever gives us the strength to stay present without fleeing from what we are experiencing. This helps us avoid feeling overwhelmed and maintain a more balanced and serene perspective.

When we learn to observe the cycle of our emotions, we can also begin to recognize recurring patterns. Perhaps we discover that certain situations always trigger the same type of emotional reaction, or that we tend to avoid certain emotions rather than face them. This awareness is a powerful tool for personal growth because it allows us to work on ourselves and transform old emotional patterns into healthier, more conscious responses.

- **Emotional cycle observation exercise**: When you feel a strong emotion, observe how it evolves over time. Take a few minutes to feel how it builds and then, gradually, begins to fade. This will help you understand that emotions are not permanent and that you can face them without being overwhelmed.

4. Emotional Intelligence: Using Emotions as a Tool for Growth

Being aware of your emotions and staying vigilant over them means developing deep emotional intelligence. Emotional intelligence is the ability to recognize, understand, and manage emotions in a way that improves our well-being and relationships. Rather than seeing emotions as uncontrollable forces or threats, we can learn to use them as valuable tools for growing and improving our lives.

When we can observe our emotions without being overwhelmed by them, we can use them as guides to make more conscious decisions. Emotions tell us what matters to us, what motivates us, and what scares us. When we learn to stay aware and vigilant of these feelings, we can make choices that are more aligned with our values and deepest needs.

Emotional intelligence also helps us improve our relationships because it enables us to better understand the emotions of others and respond with greater empathy and sensitivity. When we are aware of our own emotions, we can more easily recognize what others are feeling, creating more authentic and compassionate relationships.

- **Exercise to develop emotional intelligence**: Whenever you find yourself in an emotionally complex situation, pause and ask yourself, "How can I use this emotion to better understand myself or the other person?" This will help you see emotions not as obstacles but as opportunities for growth.

5. Presence and Connection: Staying Grounded in the Here and Now

Being aware of your emotions also means learning to stay present in the moment. Often, emotions drag us into the past or the future: we relive old wounds or worry about what might happen. But emotional awareness requires us to stay grounded in the here and now, where emotions arise and manifest.

When we are present with our emotions, we can face them with greater clarity without being consumed by anxiety or regret. Presence allows us to observe the emotion for what it is, without adding the weight of past interpretations or future projections. It is a state of connection with oneself that gives us the strength to face even the most difficult emotions with calm and serenity.

The practice of emotional awareness is thus a daily exercise in presence, in reconnecting with the body and mind, and in accepting the emotions that arise without trying to change or eliminate them. When we are present, emotions do not scare us because we know we can face them moment by moment, without being overwhelmed.

- **Emotional presence exercise**: Each day, take a few minutes to practice being present with your emotions. Sit quietly, close your eyes, and bring your attention to the sensations in your body. Observe the emotions that arise without trying to change them. This will help you develop a deeper connection with your emotional state.

Conclusion: The Power of Emotional Awareness

Staying aware and vigilant of your emotions is an act of self-love, a journey of inner discovery that leads to living with greater balance and wisdom. When we are aware of our emotions, we can use them as tools for growth, as guides to better understand our needs, desires, and limits. Instead of being swept away by emotions, we learn to dialogue with them, to observe them, and to transform them into valuable resources for our personal evolution.

Emotional awareness offers us the opportunity to live more authentically and freely, to make more conscious decisions, and to build deeper, more meaningful relationships. It is a path that requires practice and attention but, once embarked upon, allows us to navigate the sea of emotions with grace and confidence, knowing that every storm can be faced and overcome with the strength of presence and awareness.

Final Thoughts and Advice

Life is a journey of self-discovery and continuous growth, where each step brings us closer to a deeper understanding of ourselves and the world around us. The path to greater emotional awareness, the ability to love freely without dependency, and achieving emotional balance is not linear. It's a road full of highs and lows, moments of clarity, and times of confusion. Yet, in every moment, even the most difficult ones, we are given the opportunity to evolve, learn, and blossom into more authentic and self-aware individuals.

At the end of this reflective journey, one realizes that true power lies in our ability to stay present, to be vigilant over what happens within us, and to face life with an open heart and a conscious mind. Personal growth, authentic love, and emotional balance are not distant or unattainable goals but rather daily practices nurtured by our willingness to learn, change, and be kind to ourselves along the way.

1. Embrace Change as Part of the Journey

The first, and perhaps most important, piece of advice is to embrace change as an inevitable and positive part of life. Personal growth only happens when we are willing to let go of what no longer serves us and welcome new perspectives, new experiences, and new versions of ourselves. Every change, even those that initially seem painful or frightening, carries a seed of growth, a lesson that prepares us to be stronger and more self-aware.

Change is not to be feared but embraced with curiosity. Every phase of life has its lessons and challenges, and learning to navigate through them with flexibility and openness allows us to live with more ease and gratitude.

- **Advice**: Whenever you face a change, ask yourself, "What opportunity for growth is this situation offering me?" This simple shift in perspective will help you see change as an integral part of your journey.

2. Cultivate Daily Mindfulness

Mindfulness is the key to staying connected to ourselves and approaching life with greater balance. Cultivating mindfulness means being present in the moment, observing our thoughts and emotions without judgment, and learning to respond with calm and emotional intelligence. It is through mindfulness that we can recognize our deepest needs and make decisions more aligned with our values.

The practice of mindfulness doesn't require much time but does require consistency. Just a few minutes each day dedicated to reflection, meditation, or simply listening to our emotions can help us develop a deeper connection with ourselves.

- **Advice:** Dedicate 5-10 minutes each day to mindfulness practices, such as meditation or quiet reflection. Sit in a peaceful spot, close your eyes, and focus on your breath or how you feel in that moment. This will help you maintain a constant connection to your emotional and mental state.

3. Practice Self-Love as a Form of Deep Care

Self-love is the foundation of all personal growth and healthy relationships. We cannot love others freely until we learn to nourish ourselves, respect our limits, and cultivate a kind, compassionate relationship with our inner self. This means caring for our emotional, physical, and mental well-being without waiting for someone else to do it for us.

Self-love requires self-compassion during tough times, the courage to say "no" when necessary, and the ability to celebrate our successes without belittling ourselves. The more we learn to take care of ourselves, the more we realize how important it is to do the same in our relationships with others, to avoid emotional dependency and create bonds based on respect and reciprocity.

- **Advice:** Every day, take a moment to do something that deeply nourishes you. It could be a walk in nature, a creative activity, or simply resting. Remember that you deserve care and attention, just like the people you love.

4. Develop the Ability to Let Go

Learning to let go is one of life's hardest lessons but also one of the most liberating. Much of our suffering comes from attachment to people, situations, or expectations that we cannot control. Letting go does not mean giving up or not caring but accepting that some things are beyond our control and that life requires us to release what no longer serves us to make space for the new.

This ability is essential for living free and authentic love, where we don't seek to possess or hold onto the other but allow them to be themselves in their evolution. It's also fundamental for our emotional well-being: holding onto old pains, grudges, or regrets prevents us from fully living in the present.

- **Advice**: When facing a situation you cannot change, practice the art of letting go. Ask yourself, "What can I do to accept what I can't control and focus on what I can change?" This will help you live with more lightness and serenity.

5. Make Gratitude a Daily Practice

Gratitude is one of the most powerful practices for maintaining emotional balance and cultivating a positive outlook on life. Often, we focus on what we lack, what's not going well, or what we want to achieve, forgetting all that we already have. Gratitude brings us back to the present, reminding us of the small and great blessings that fill our lives and allowing us to appreciate each moment for what it is.

Practicing gratitude doesn't mean denying difficulties but being able to see the beauty that exists alongside them. Each day is an opportunity to find something to be grateful for, even in the darkest moments. This helps us cultivate a more open, trusting, and peaceful heart.

- **Advice**: Every night before going to bed, take a moment to reflect on three things you are grateful for during the day. They could be small gestures, meaningful encounters, or simply the beauty of a moment lived. Gratitude will help you end the day with a sense of fullness and contentment.

Conclusion: Life as an Opportunity for Evolution

In conclusion, life is a continuous opportunity for evolution and transformation. Every day offers us the chance to learn something new, to grow, and to become more aware of ourselves and others. The key to living with fullness and serenity lies in staying present, cultivating gratitude, loving ourselves and others freely and authentically, and accepting change as a natural part of our journey.

Remaining vigilant over our emotions, developing emotional intelligence, and learning to love without dependence are practices that allow us to face life with balance, inner strength, and a heart always open to the beauty and opportunities that each day brings.

Personal growth has no end—it is an infinite journey. And that is its greatest gift: it reminds us that, no matter our story, we can always evolve, learn, improve, and live with greater authenticity and fullness.